Matilda Heindow

The Art of Feeling Better

How I heal my
mental health
(and you can too)

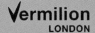

Vermilion
LONDON

For all the people who love me as I am,
and through it all

Vermilion, an imprint of Ebury Publishing,
20 Vauxhall Bridge Road,
London SW1V 2SA

Vermilion is part of the Penguin Random House group of companies
whose addresses can be found at global.penguinrandomhouse.com

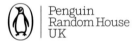

Penguin
Random House
UK

First published by Vermilion in 2023

www.penguin.co.uk

A CIP catalogue record for this book is available from the British Library

ISBN 9781785044090

Printed and bound in China by C&C Offset Printing Co., Ltd.

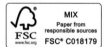

MIX
Paper from
responsible sources
FSC® C018179

Penguin Random House is committed to a sustainable future for our
business, our readers and our planet. This book is made from Forest
Stewardship Council® certified paper.

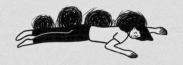

CONTENTS

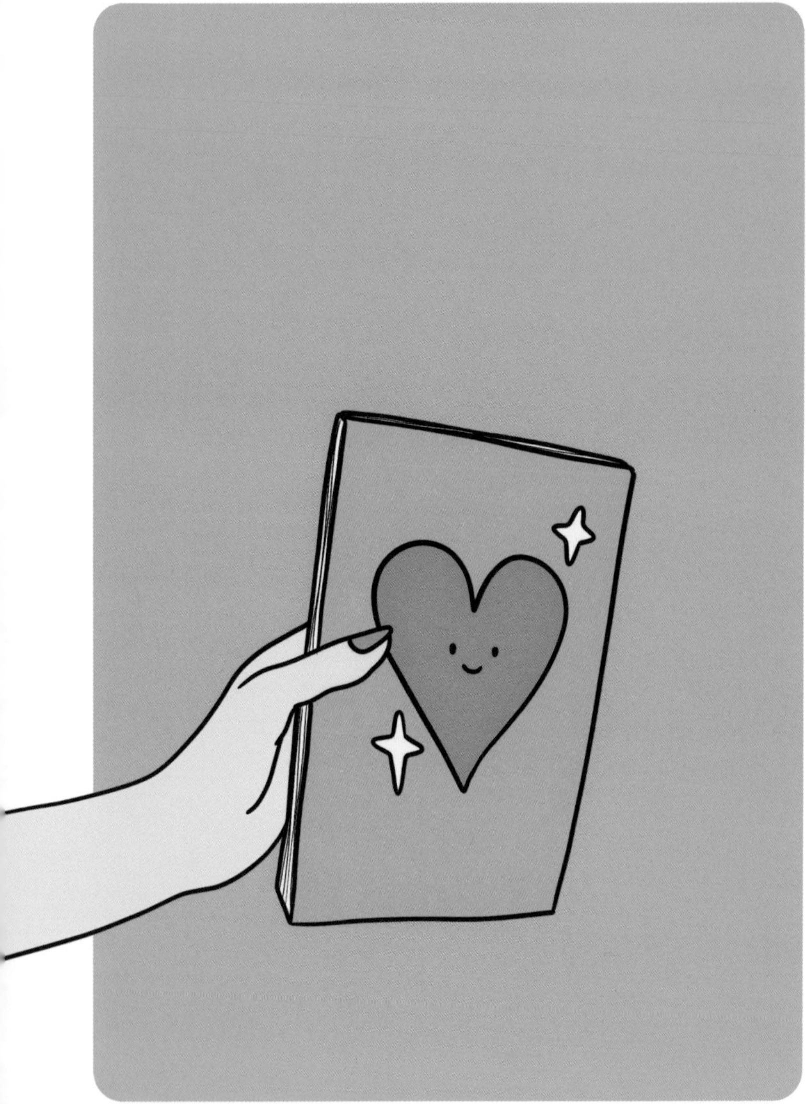

INTRODUCTION:
This book is for you

I wrote this book for you – yes, you. Perhaps it was a gift from someone who loves you, or maybe it was a gift to yourself. You might have picked it up because you've struggled with your mental health, or are struggling right now, or maybe you haven't felt like yourself in a long time. You might be feeling hopeful or hopeless. Whoever you are, whatever you are going through, you have mental health to look after, so this book is for you.

This book chronicles my own mental health battles, from the first symptom and the first therapy visit to the positive place I'm in now – an honest recovery journey scattered with highs and lows, setbacks and victories and everything I learnt along the way. I wrote it because as common as my experience is, very few people talk about their mental health struggles. I have used my experience as a starting point to speak to you about your mental health and what you may go through too, in the past, present or future. I want to show you that, even in your own low moments, you are far from alone and you are certainly not lost. Your highs are on the horizon.

In these pages I describe what I've learnt on my journey (and what I've unlearned). In pictures and words, I share the tips I've picked up along the way that have made it possible to heal, the self-care tools that can truly help, the coping mechanisms that can provide a life raft on the road to recovery and the new perspectives that come when you make friends with yourself again. In short, I share how I learned to thrive (not just survive), so you can take from my experience anything that's useful for you.

This book covers sensitive topics including suicide, trauma and grief. Do not feel obligated to read anything that might feel too heavy for you right now. Those parts are there because I want to share the realities of my journey, and I believe these topics shouldn't be taboo. Those sections will be there for you when you're ready to read them, and they are marked with this symbol:

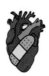

I invite you to read this book however you need, whether that is from start to finish or dipping into the sections that might help you at a difficult time. Each chapter is short and accompanied by my illustrations, so I hope it will be easy for you to take from it what you need, when you need it. I encourage you to highlight and scribble in the pages that speak to you, to lend this book to a friend who hasn't been feeling good lately or keep it close by for those moments when you need it most. I would love for you to use it in whatever way most helps you and your loved ones.

I hope this book can be a reminder that there are millions of people who have felt similarly to you and that there are hundreds of ways to heal. My greatest wish is to provide you with a little hope whatever you're going through – like a hand holding yours, even when the world feels like it's collapsing around you. The perspectives, tips and tricks in these pages may help even when you aren't sure what you need, or when you don't have enough energy to know where to start. Use what speaks to you and leave aside the rest for another day.

Most of all, I hope this book serves as a reminder to look after your mental health and treat yourself like someone worth taking care of – because you are.

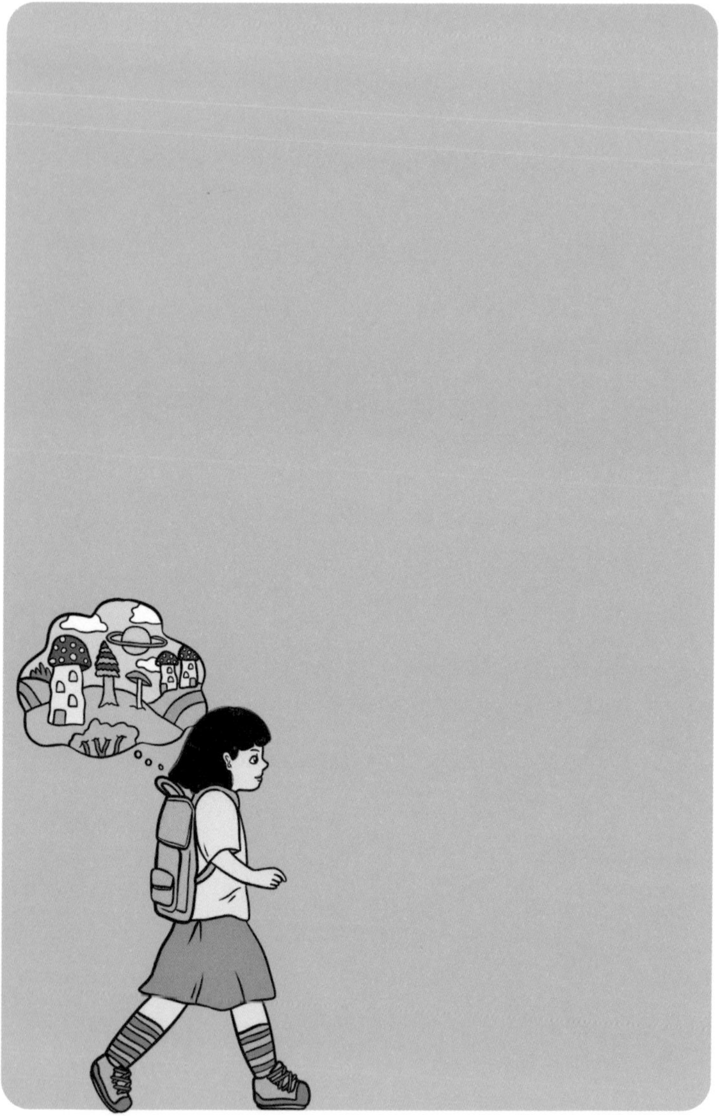

Mental illness and me

I can't remember exactly when I first started feeling like there was something wrong with me. I suspect that feeling was there for a long time.

My mum tells me I was extremely easy-going as a baby – perfectly content and calm most of the time. It made her wonder what all the fuss of parenting was all about. I learned to talk and I never stopped talking. My favourite thing to do was to ask my grandparents questions about absolutely everything. I loved their old handbound books, which they would lift down from the shelves to answer my many questions. I had a rich inner life; I would tell myself stories that built into complex internal worlds, with imaginary people, places and events that overlapped and expanded over years of daydreaming. In my early life, my mind was a sacred space that I loved inhabiting. How things change.

The more I saw of the world, the more new experiences I encountered, the more wary and fearful I became. Those feelings intensified in school. Most other children seemed free of worry, but I was too nervous to even climb trees with them. I would often cry quietly in the middle of third-grade math class because I didn't understand a single thing. I got my first nose-bleed in that class; I hid my face in my hands, too embarrassed to draw attention to myself. When the teacher asked me to put my hands down, the blood had smeared onto my face and palms, sticky and thick. I was intensely ashamed. I was later diagnosed with dyscalculia, a learning disability that makes number comprehension very difficult, as well as ADHD which makes concentrating in general rather tricky too, unless I am interested in the topic.

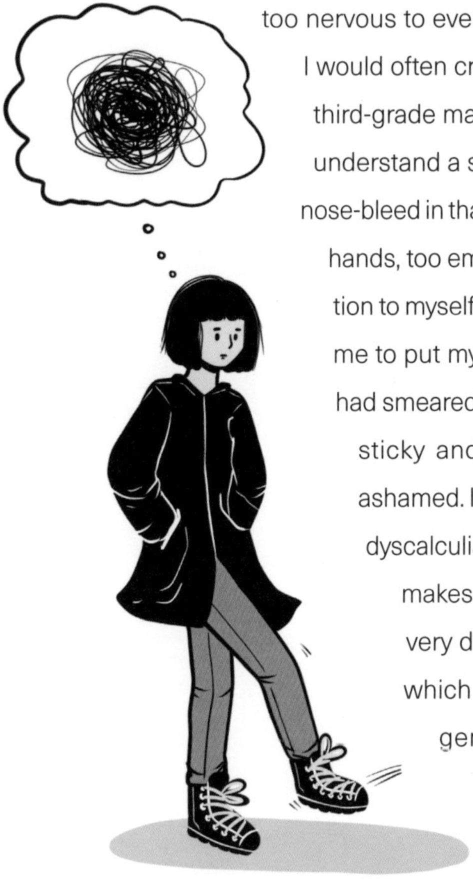

I felt I was 'wrong' – partly because I was told so. Adults chastized me constantly for being too sensitive and for not trying hard enough in school. It upset me, because I was trying as hard as I humanly could – and it wasn't enough. By the age of 14, I was consumed by anxiety and something else I couldn't quite explain. I noticed I didn't experience curiosity, joy or contentment anymore. I wasn't sure when that had stopped, but by that point I don't think I cared. I was a teenager and teens are supposed to be hormonal and full of angst, right?

But this didn't feel like the usual teen angst. It felt more like the part of my brain responsible for happiness had been surgically removed. I experienced prolonged periods of utter disinterest and despair – a dissonance between me and everything else.

I drafted several wills in my diary but I never asked myself why. I didn't own anything important anyway – like a house or a car – so they weren't even useful, but it felt like a thing I needed to do. My moods disturbed my parents, who were growing increasingly worried as I withdrew further into myself.

When I was 12 or 13, my mum booked me an appointment with a therapist. Her office was bright and cluttered with low-lit plants; a bowl of fidget toys sat on a little table along with a freshly opened pack of tissues with one stick-

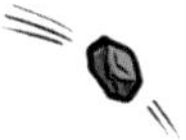

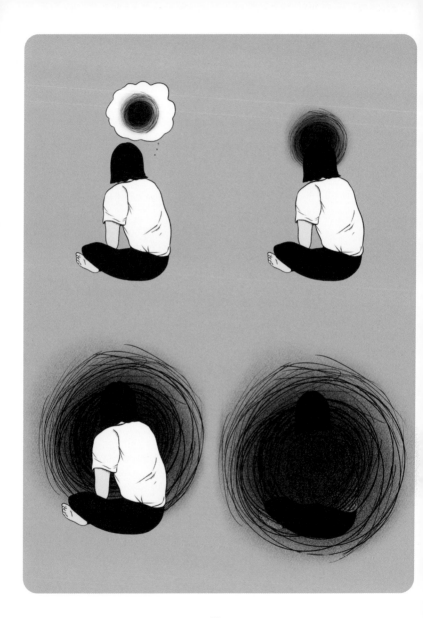

ing out slightly, like an invitation or a reminder to use it. The walls were lined with white IKEA shelves with neatly arranged psychology books and a big Matisse print in a frame.

I asked if she was allowed to choose her office art herself and she told me that nobody had asked her that before. She was quite 'matter-of-fact', in a way that made me feel uneasy, but when I asked her things like that, things that amused her, she became a little warmer. She asked me to fill out forms about depression and asked me personal questions about my home life. She asked me if I wanted to die. I didn't want to die, or at least I hadn't considered it, despite drafting the wills.

She wondered if I had been depressed for a long time and I explained that it came in waves.

'Do you experience moments of happiness?' she asked.
I never thought long about the questions before answering.
'Yes, some days I'm so happy,' I said, 'it almost feels like too much, but it never lasts. I always get depressed again.'

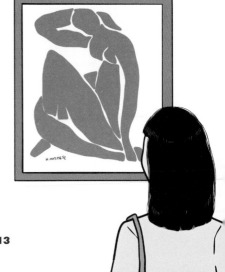

This made her pause, like a lightbulb turned on in her mind, and she scribbled something in her notebook at a speed I hadn't seen from her before. She started asking how long I'd get happy for, if I slept less then, if I became impulsive or spoke fast during these days of happiness. She made me fill out new forms, did more in-depth psychological evaluations and told me she suspected bipolar disorder. I didn't know exactly what that was, only that it was probably bad.

Later that night I googled 'bipolar disorder'. Afterwards, I cried hard into my pillow until I had a headache and the pillowcase had an imprint of my wet eyeliner. I cried because I knew she was right, and I knew that my life had changed forever. A few weeks later it was confirmed and I was referred to a bipolar and psychosis unit. I had a team composed of a doctor, therapist, psychiatrist, occupational therapist, caseworker and nurse. They put me on medications that had long, unpronounceable names. The medications gave me

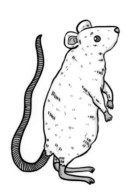

vertigo and shaky hands and rashes and auditory hallucinations right before bed, but they also made me less moody, which was the point.

I felt like a science experiment, like my youth and privacy were being taken from me – like a person who was sick, worrying everyone. I was still as 'wrong' as I was before, but now the wrongness had names like bipolar and generalized anxiety and social anxiety and panic disorder, and I was 'hard to treat' because of the complex comorbidity of disorders all playing off of each other.

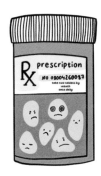

Looking back, it was a huge adjustment that felt like the end of everything. I was grieving the previous versions of me; I was aching for the chilled-out baby version of me, or the inquisitive toddler version of me, or even the obliviously depressed 13-year-old me.

The 'me' I am now wishes I could go back and tell myself that I was never wrong or bad or defective. The 'me' I am now has learnt so much from those difficult days – about myself and about how each of us needs to look after our mental health. To not be consumed by my darkest thoughts and heaviest feelings, but to let them inform me of what needs to change or adapt or process. To not give into the little voice that sometimes tells me to give up, but to find ways to prove it wrong. My recovery started as a slow reprogramming of my mind, dissecting and looking deeply into the parts that I pushed aside for so long. It was about finding the courage to endure the healing process, as I endured living with mental illness for so long.

I wish I could put this book into the little hands of my younger self and say, 'Look at what you've learnt! Look at what you can do when you cheer yourself on. Look at this version of yourself – she loves you!'

When I was twenty, I started an Instagram account where I scribbled about my struggles with mental health and the lessons I'd learned trying to make sense of what was happening. It was cathartic, and I hoped my drawings would reach someone who struggled like I did. It became my safe little corner of the internet, and to my surprise, it grew fast. Apparently, hundreds of thousands of people could relate. I was met with comments like, 'It's like I wrote this!' or, 'You put into words something I felt but didn't know how to explain'. Seeing that made me realize that my story wasn't as unique as I'd thought. So, I continued sharing it, and I found a purpose – to help others and help change how we view mental illness.

My illness used to be my biggest limitation – the reason I felt like I didn't fit in anywhere – but it has propelled me in a new direction, one that motivated me to get better so I can show other people that it's possible. I thought my vulnerability and sensitivity were weaknesses – turns out they are superpowers. Now I spend most of my days in a little apartment in Stockholm, making my art, working to raise awareness of mental health, feeling and healing – soaking in the light that I didn't think I'd ever feel, and moving through the world a little lighter day-by-day. Some days are still dark, but that darkness doesn't swallow me anymore, because I have trained the muscles necessary to pull myself up again.

At my worst, I didn't think it would ever get better. Today, I have days where I wake up with a heart full of joy and excitement. Inside this little book, I have written about some of the things that make this possible for me.

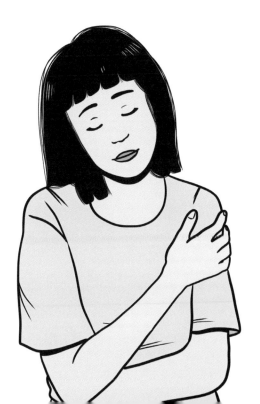

Chapter 1

'IS THERE SOMETHING WRONG WITH ME?' (NO)

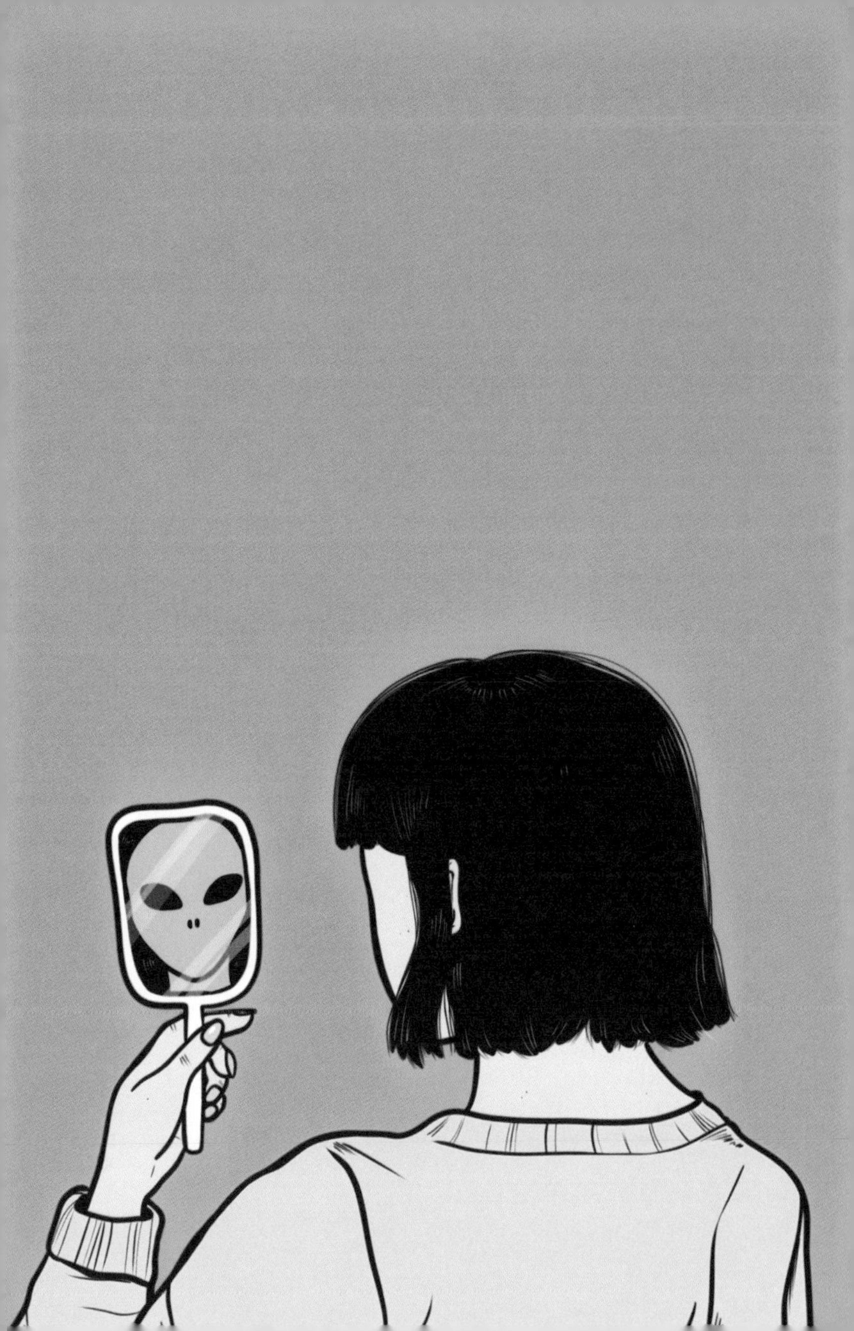

'What's happening to me?'

Let's take a moment to check in: how are you feeling right now? Maybe you picked up this book because you feel something is wrong with you, or you're worried about someone close to you. I want to reassure you that you are not alone in these feelings and there's nothing weird about what you're going through. Take a big breath, stretch out your legs, unclench your jaw and get comfortable. Are you ready?

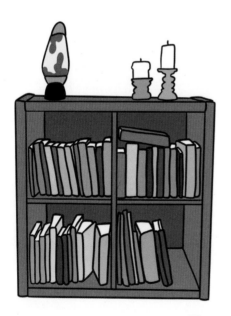

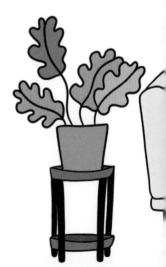

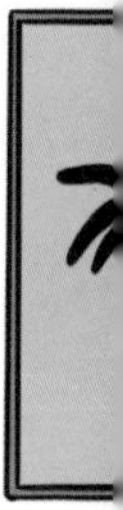

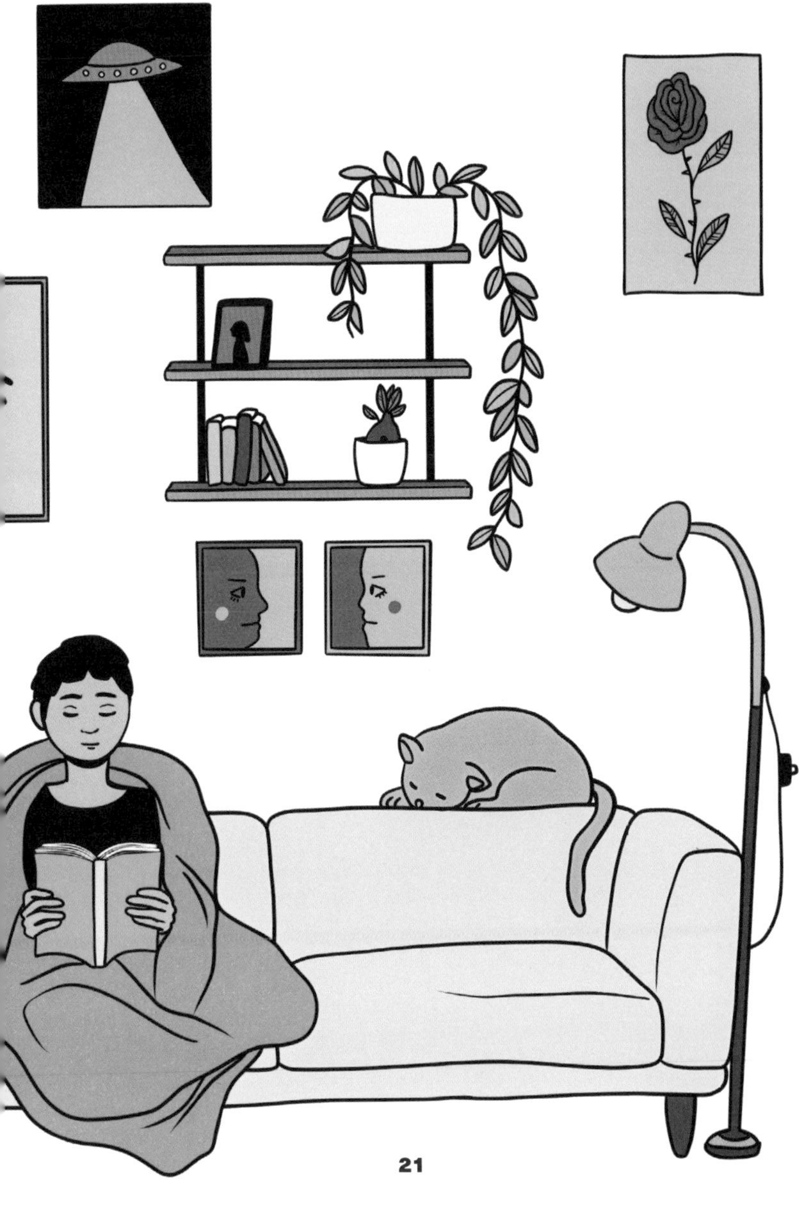

Before my therapist said the words 'bipolar disorder', I thought I was 'too sensitive' and 'too moody'. Acknowledging what was really going on opened up my understanding of how I could help myself, with the right support. The feelings and thoughts that surround you when you're struggling with your mental health can be confusing. You may not understand that you have a problem and that help is out there for you.

Anybody could struggle with their mental health, and anybody could develop a mental illness. So how can we tell when 'normal' sadness or stress have become a bigger problem? The first step is knowing the common signs of declining mental health. The sooner we notice this, the easier it will be to work through what we're feeling.

inability to carry out daily activities

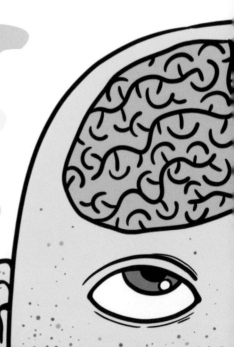

changes in mood, sleep, or eating habits

inability to cope with everyday stress

excessive worry or fear

feeling sad

See the signs below and ask yourself:

- Are you finding it hard to cope with everyday stress?
- Has your sleep changed?
- Are you eating differently?
- Are you finding it harder to concentrate?
- Are you withdrawing from social activities?

I know how difficult it can be in the moment, especially if this is the first time you're going through it, but acknowledging the early warning signs is your first step towards feeling better.

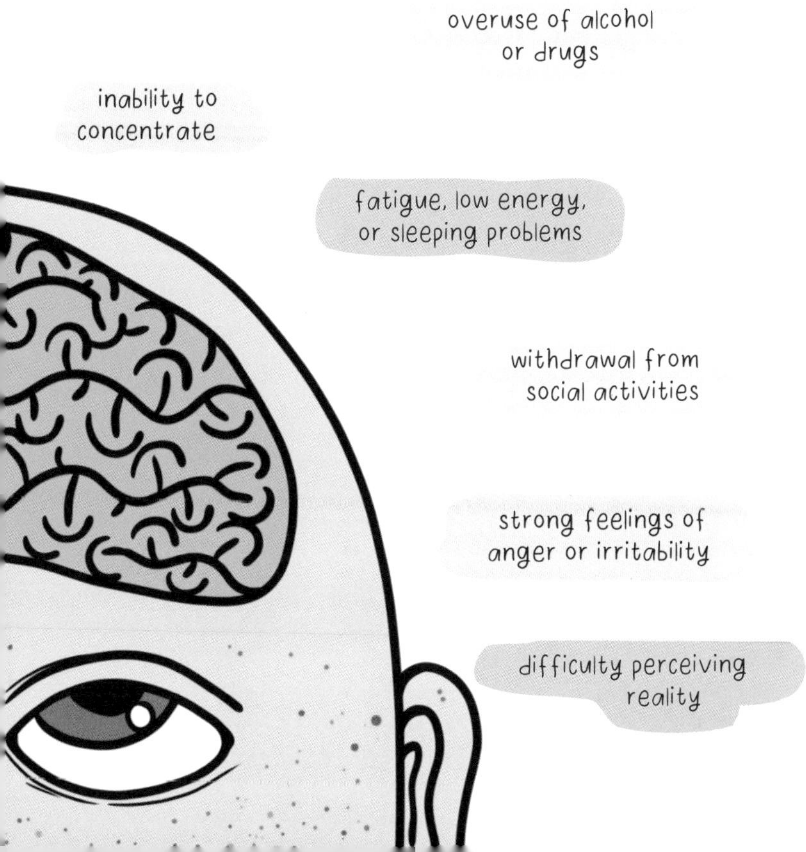
overuse of alcohol or drugs
inability to concentrate
fatigue, low energy, or sleeping problems
withdrawal from social activities
strong feelings of anger or irritability
difficulty perceiving reality

We all have 'mental health'

We all have mental health; it is the sum total of our psychological, emotional and social wellbeing. Tending to it is vital, but often isn't prioritized. I believe it's because most of us were not properly taught to do so.

When I first got sick, I felt like a failure, but I realized recently that I was failed by a world that isn't accessible to those of us with disabilities or illnesses. I wonder how different my life would have been if I didn't have to deal with the disorganisation and executive dysfunction of ADHD, or the whirlwind of my mood disorder. Many of us don't have access to mental health resources and treatment, many of

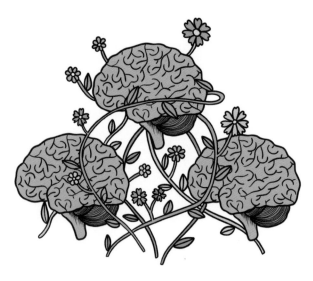

us grew up in homes and within communities where mental health problems were stigmatized, where questions or worries or warning signs remained unaddressed. I think society isn't exactly set up to nurture our collective mental health, but instead often makes it worse.

Not too long after my first set of diagnoses, I watched a lot of friends develop problems in high school: kids getting burnt-out or strung-out at the age of 16, going to inpatient facilities or switching schools because the pressure was too much. Since then, I have seen colleagues at work break down from stress, having to take extended sick leaves. Many people I've met have had skewed, negative relationships with their bodies and some form of disordered eating. Poor mental health, in some form, isn't that unusual.

Between genetics, generational trauma, unequal societies, poor working conditions, high academic expectations, lack of access to healthcare, and stress, it's not surprising that so many of us struggle with our mental health. So let us never forget: if you experience problems or struggles with your mental health, it is not your fault.

The rhythm of our daily lives doesn't always leave room for us to tend to our emotional wellbeing. In between obligations and responsibilities it can be hard to find time for self-nurturing. But to simply set aside a moment each day to perform a therapeutic exercise, do a mindfulness activity, or check in with your feelings, forms a habit that can strengthen mental health, even on good days. The state of our mental health is fluid and can change rapidly – to create a solid set of coping tools builds a foundation we can fall back on when we're struggling. Trying different self-help strategies and finding ones that work for you is like decorating a living space, building it piece by piece until you've got places to rest, to create, to converse, and to move your body in ways that are comfortable to you. Your brain is your permanent inner home, so furnishing it according to your own needs really makes a difference.

What mental illness feels like

Even though we have diagnostic manuals for mental illness, the way each person experiences mental distress can never fit into any one box. It's as individual as our fingerprints; our unique experiences are shaped by nurture, culture and daily life. But the one thing every mental health disorder has in common is that it negatively impacts our day-to-day life. One in four people will at some point in their lives experience a mental health condition, but everyone has mental health, which can decline or increase, just like our physical health. Looking after our mental health can help us prevent mental illness in the long term.

For me, mental illness can shrink and stunt everything. The sicker I am, the more limitations and hurdles appear, and the bigger the distance grows between me and everyone else. Small tasks become impossible feats, and my energy gets sucked out of me like a balloon slowly deflating. Hobbies become stressors or feel like too much effort. It feels like losing myself little by little, in constant anticipation of impending doom. It feels like blowing out the candles on your birthday cake and wishing that you could just go to bed. Pulling from my mixed bag of comorbid conditions, there's been paranoia, catastrophizing, delusion, despair, hopelessness, numbness, traumatic stress, racing thoughts – sometimes on a loop that seems never-ending.

Some people really underestimate the immeasurable toll mental illness can take on someone. I say it's like getting stuck in quicksand; it's not the drowning that gets you, it is the sheer exhaustion of trying to pull yourself out that wears you down.

To survive, like in quicksand, you must lean back, lean into it, even though it's scary. Then, call for help, and accept the helping hands of others. Doing that can help you stay afloat, even when it feels like you'll hit the bottom.

I sat in quicksand for years, feeling crushed, until I had enough help to lift me out: coping techniques, human connections and strength. Sometimes a foot slips back in, but each time it gets a little easier to pull myself out again.

MY DEPRESSION FEELS LIKE

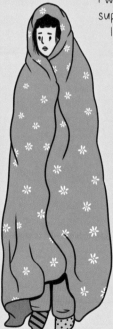

i want to do new things but i don't have the energy

i want to ask for support but i feel like a burden

i want to work on myself to become better but it feels too hopeless

i want to do things i like but nothing gets me excited or feels good anymore

i want to believe it will get better but i struggle to imagine that possibility

i want to get things done but i have no motivation

i want to feel loved by others but i don't feel like i'm even likeable

i want to be happy but what's the point?

i'm not happy here

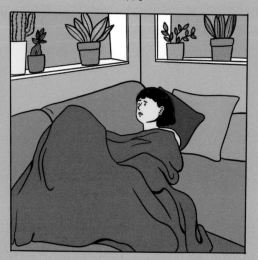

i'm not happy here either

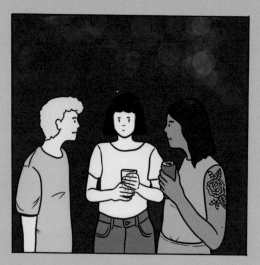

i'm still not happy here

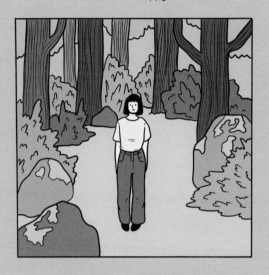

why am i not happy here?

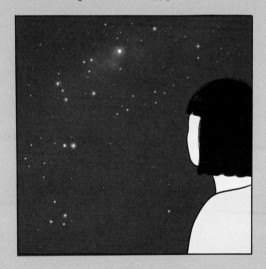

What mental illness looks like

Sometimes when I open up about my experience with anxiety and depression, I am met by puzzled looks, eyes scanning me up and down, and a frown: 'Oh, I wouldn't have guessed that, you don't look anxious. You don't seem depressed.' A good first impression is important to me, and I've had years to play pretend-happy, working hard to make other people feel safe and happy in my social circle. Anxiety can be perceived as disinterest or shyness, depression can be hidden quite easily with a simple 'I'm just tired, I didn't get much sleep'. Since mental illness is made up of disordered thoughts and behaviours behind closed doors, it can go unnoticed to others. Not only is it invisible in many ways, it's also often purposefully hidden away because we fear what other people might think about us if we're honest.

To those who aren't informed about mental health, mental illness can be synonymous to weak, damaged, dramatic, attention-seeking, or dangerous. I opened up about my bipolar disorder to one employer, but I later quit that job due to a toxic work environment. Said employer later gave me a call to let me know that he'd wanted to fire me but didn't because I might 'off-myself', like his friend with bipolar disorder tragically did. After that I never divulged my health to people at work. The way my former employer saw me changed drastically, even though nothing had changed about me at all. I was just as competent as before, but he let his own preconceptions warp his perception of me.

Preconceptions about mental illness are huge hurdles to normalizing mental health. To be open with our struggles we need to feel as though we will be received with empathy, and not with fear or prejudice. He probably didn't know many people with bipolar disorder, because if he did, he would know that we are not that rare. The more people you meet with different lives and experiences, the more we learn about how different brains work, the more accepting we will be of everyone's differences. It can be scary to open up, but once we have safe people around us who we can talk to and rely upon, it can really help others to understand that mental illness isn't some scary elephant in the room, but something to be talked about, because it can happen to anyone.

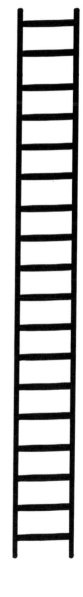

DEPRESSION CAN LOOK LIKE

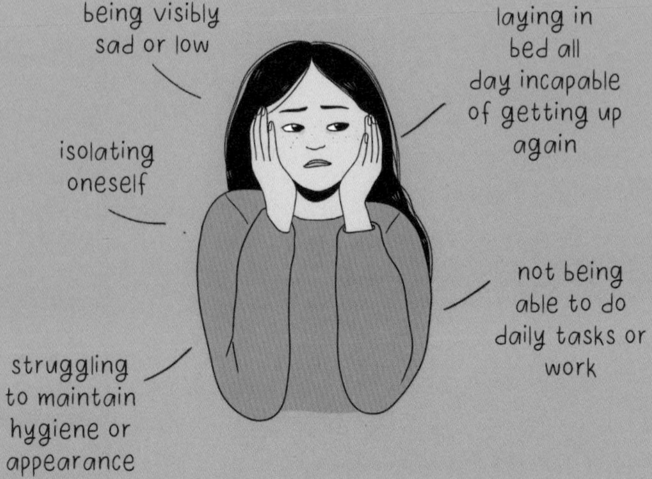
being visibly sad or low
laying in bed all day incapable of getting up again
isolating oneself
not being able to do daily tasks or work
struggling to maintain hygiene or appearance

AND ALSO LIKE

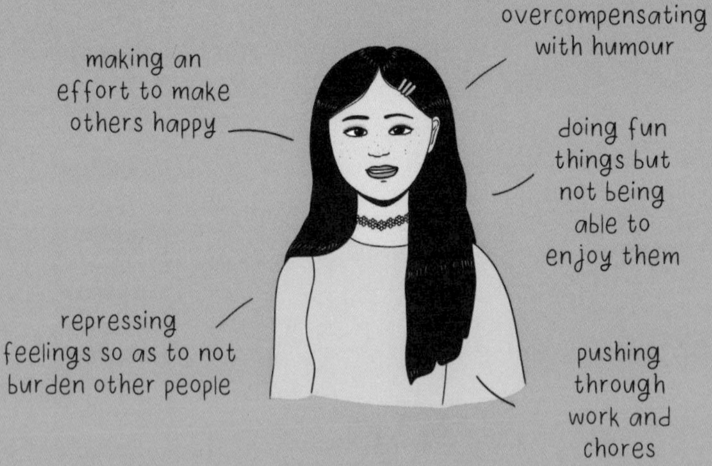
overcompensating with humour
making an effort to make others happy
doing fun things but not being able to enjoy them
repressing feelings so as to not burden other people
pushing through work and chores

ANXIETY CAN LOOK LIKE

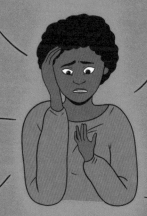

being socially awkward and fearful of social interaction
having intense panic attacks
seeming insecure
withdrawing from activities involving others
being shy and quiet

AND ALSO LIKE

having anxiety attacks that are internal and go unnoticed
overcompensating socially to fit ir
distracting yourself with escapism because sitting with your thoughts feels unbearable
avoiding things and situations that trigger anxiety as often as possible

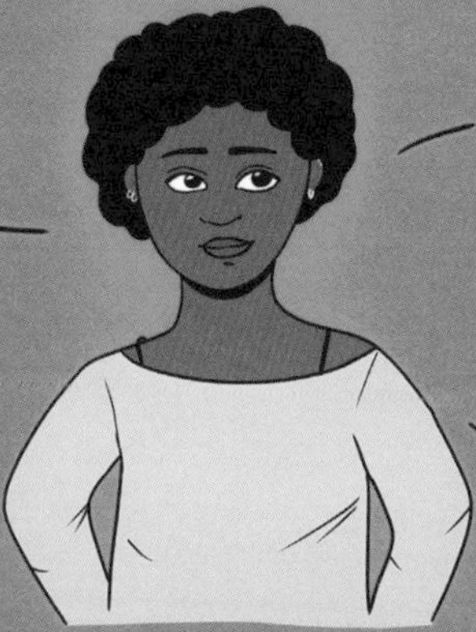

What's going on for you?

When someone asks you how you're feeling, do you find yourself instinctively saying 'I'm fine', when really you are far from it?

Opportunities to reveal your honest feelings can be few and far between. Being honest about our negative feelings can feel like a faux pas. A support system is pivotal for healing. Think about who you could invite to be part of yours – a friend, an online group, a counsellor, your guardian or relatives, a colleague who is going through something similar, perhaps? Building connections with other people makes a huge difference. Sometimes we even lie to ourselves: we push away our feelings because they are too painful and we've got so much other stuff that needs to get done. Before we know it, we've been walking around with unresolved pain, carrying it everywhere, each step getting a little heavier.

So, how are you really feeling? There are no wrong answers, nothing too vulnerable or unspeakable. How are you, right now at this moment?

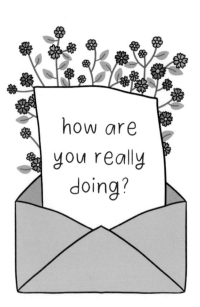

how are you really doing?

ask yourself:

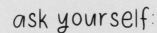

what weighs on me right now?

are there feelings that i have been repressing?

do i feel shame or guilt right now, for any reason?

are there things that happened in the past that really hurt and rattle me when i'm reminded of them?

am i carrying my worry as tenseness in my body right now, and if so, where?

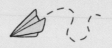

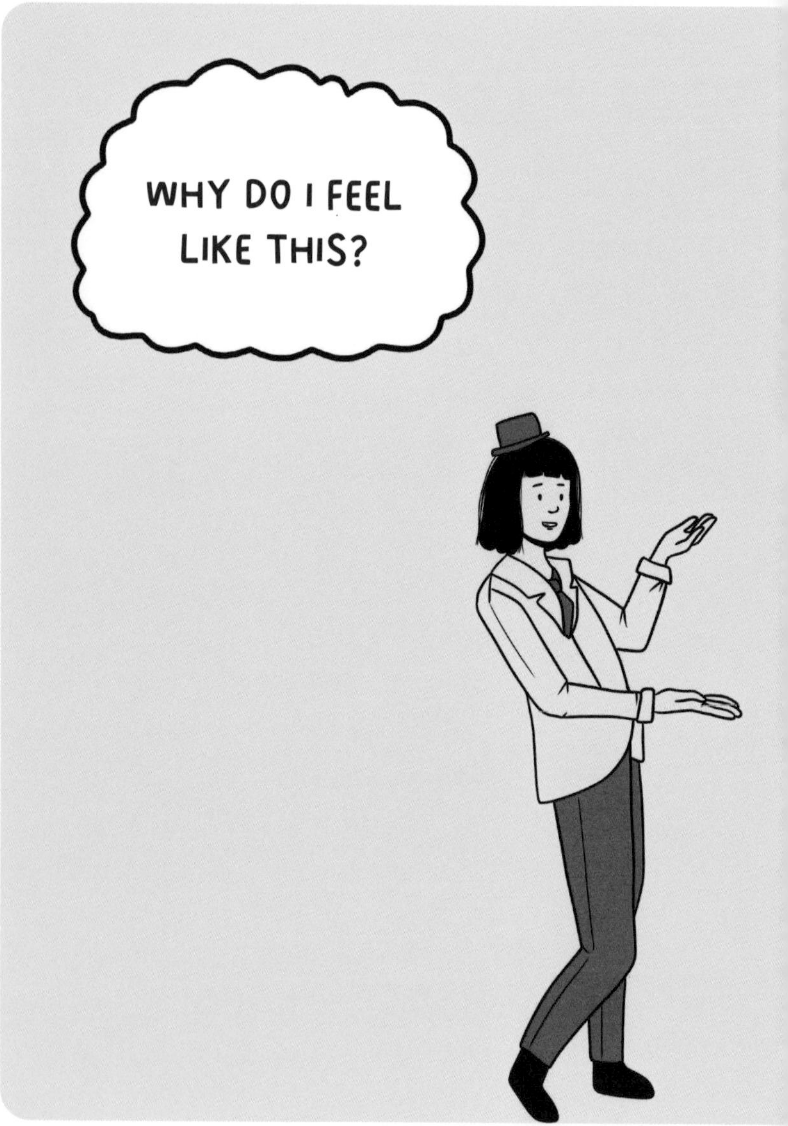
WHY DO I FEEL LIKE THIS?

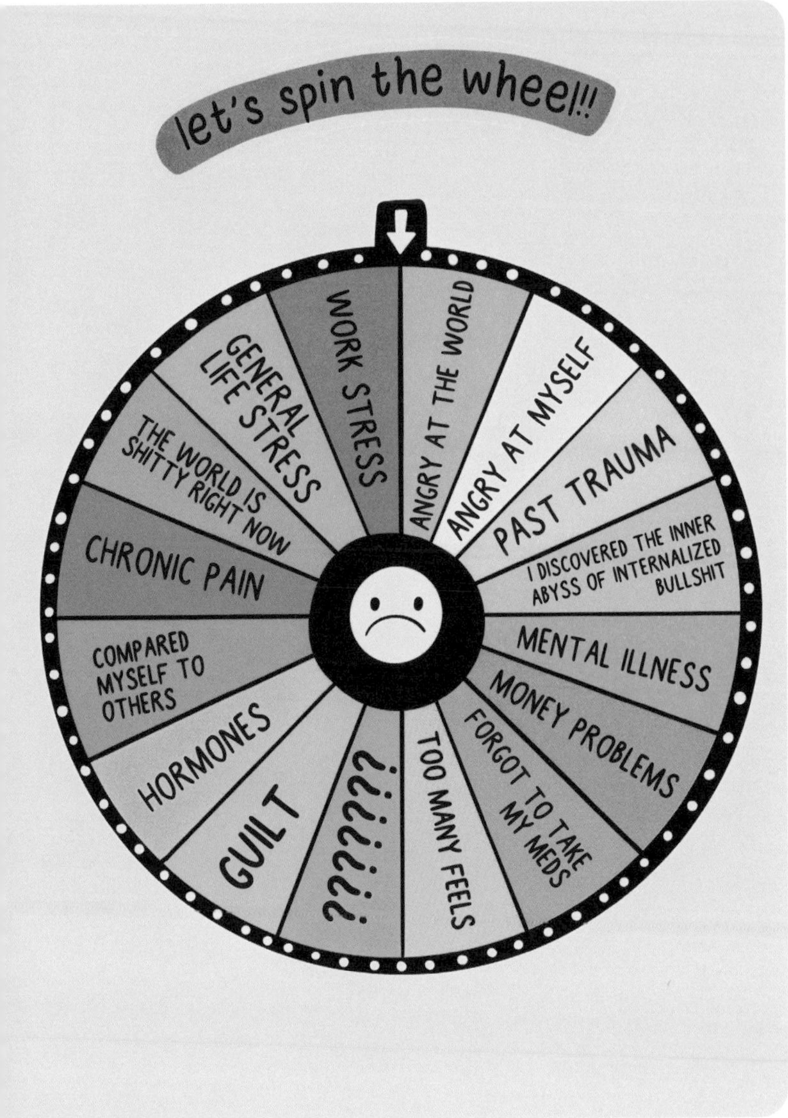
let's spin the wheel!!!
WORK STRESS
ANGRY AT THE WORLD
ANGRY AT MYSELF
PAST TRAUMA
I DISCOVERED THE INNER ABYSS OF INTERNALIZED BULLSHIT
MENTAL ILLNESS
MONEY PROBLEMS
FORGOT TO TAKE MY MEDS
TOO MANY FEELS
¿¿¿¿???
GUILT
HORMONES
COMPARED MYSELF TO OTHERS
CHRONIC PAIN
THE WORLD IS SHITTY RIGHT NOW
GENERAL LIFE STRESS

It's okay to ask for help

The beginning of my mental health journey can be described in just one word: overwhelming. Something is wrong: now what? Where do I go? What do I say? What will happen? These are the questions that teenage me had to grapple with.

Asking for support, even when you need it most, can be hard for a lot of reasons. You may feel scared of the response you'll get, or how you might be perceived; you may find it hard to admit you need help, or just feel confused and worried. Asking for help can be uncomfortable, because it requires us to show our vulnerability and relinquish control. We don't want to be seen as needy – we'd rather be independent and capable – but we humans are a bit needy.

i feel really overwhelmed by my messy house right now, can you come over and help me get started? i'll get us dinner afterwards!

my therapist said i should take more walks and i feel really unmotivated. do you want to come along?

this is confusing me, could you explain this to me? you're so good at making sense of things.

could i vent to you for a bit? i'd love some support

i am struggling and i need help. would you mind helping me look for mental health ressources?

We need others – support and social connection sits at the foundation of our human needs. Life can be overwhelming and, if we're not feeling good, simple tasks like doing the dishes or booking an appointment can feel close to impossible. The good news is most people like helping others.

It's best not to ask by opening the conversation with a version of 'I feel terrible for asking', because there's no reason to feel guilty. Our society might praise self-reliance, but we cannot go through life successfully without practicing our ability to let others help us and, in turn, to help others. Help can come in many forms: sometimes you might want a listening ear, other times you might benefit from practical advice or help with daily tasks.

You might have asked your friends, family or partner for help and realized that what you really need is a professional. Don't be afraid of taking that first step of reaching out to your doctor or to a therapist; you don't have to know what to say or know what's going to happen. They can help you figure all of that out.

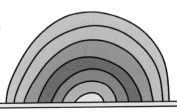

IF YOU CAN'T AFFORD THERAPY

You might find help through:
- Health insurance or your local health services
- Online therapy or counselling sessions (many therapists offer discounted rates for online-only sessions)
- Your workplace Employee Assistance Program (EAP) or your school/ university (and if you're a student check if nearby therapists offer a student discount)
- Mental health organisations and charities
- Your place of worship, if you go to one

And if none of these options pan out, seek as much advice as you can from friends, family, doctors and reliable resources online, in books and apps.

'I want to live, but I don't want to exist right now'

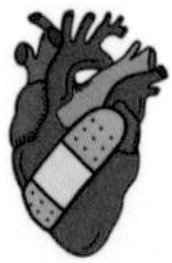

The following pages include a discussion of suicidal feelings and my suicide attempt. This is a topic I feel it's important to talk about, but if this isn't something you can manage right now, skip to page 48.

When I'm going through a rough patch, or when I'm feeling overwhelmed with big, difficult feelings, I like to imagine how nice it would be to fall into a long, anaesthetic sleep. To lay unconscious and paralyzed and unaware of not only my emotional pain, but also my very existence as a perceivable person. Everything could pause and when I wake up again, I'd be rested and warm, and there would be a palpable distance between whatever was wrong before and my current reality. But, of course, that isn't really possible, and it's not what would actually help.

Talk of suicide makes a lot of people uncomfortable. There's fear and misunderstanding around it. There's a general perception that suicide is a choice – that suicidal people want to die. But in actuality, in most cases, I believe it's not about wishing to die, but wanting to escape a suffering that feels all-consuming and inescapable. I believe words like 'selfish' and 'choice' need to be eradicated from discussions about suicide, because it's not a debate about morals or personal responsibility. Suicide is one of the leading causes of death, so the way we talk about it is so important.

I've had my own experience with suicide. Seventeen was a difficult age for me, and everything

MYTHS	FACTS
talking about suicide might encourage people who feel suicidal to attempt	talking about suicide is important and shows others that you are there to help and listen
suicide only happens to people with severe mental health disorders	many suicides are triggered by stressful life events and can happen to anyone
people who want to die will find a way to do so no matter what we do	suicidal feelings are often temporary and intervention can save lives
people who say they feel suicidal are seeking attention	attention-seeking behaviour should be seen as care-seeking behaviour, and be taken seriously

shattered when I was prescribed a medication that gave me drug-induced psychosis, leading to a manic episode. It started with feelings of paranoia and unreality, then it escalated to intense persecutory delusions that had me fearing for my life, thinking someone or something was about to harm me at every moment. Seeing dark shapes and shadows in the corner of my eye, feeling as if a long-clawed hand would reach out and grab me. The mania made me appear happy and motivated but, inside my head, everything was pure chaos. I didn't seek help because I was scared that I'd be taken somewhere against my will, and also because reaching out meant verbalising that this was in fact happening – something I didn't want to even admit to myself. If this happened to me now,

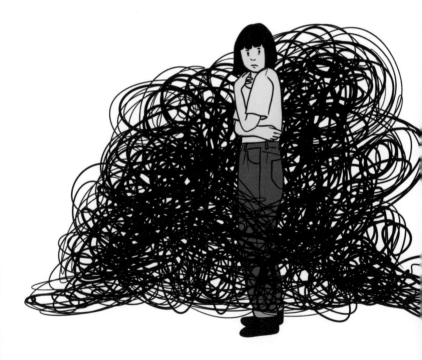

I would reach out and seek help, but I didn't understand that my psychosis was an actual medical emergency, and I didn't know how to advocate for myself at that time.

One night it got so bad, and I was so sleep deprived, I took all my medication for the next couple of weeks at once. From this point, my remaining memory of the night appears in brief flashes, fuzzy and fragmented. Two police officers found me on the side of the road by a graveyard, barefoot and incoherent, and hurried me to hospital. My vision was outlined by a black edge that was growing bigger and bigger, and as it grew a feeling of doom set in. I was propped up in a bed and fed activated coal, which absorbs poison from your stomach. My most vivid memory is the taste of the coal and how it felt in my throat going down, all clumpy and coarse.

When I woke up, I noticed I had an IV in my arm, then I saw my family lingering by my hospital bed, pale faces, more pained than I had ever seen them before, making my gut wrench. When I saw myself in the mirror for the first time in the adjacent bathroom, I didn't recognize myself. The activated coal had dried into the corners of my mouth and in between my gums, my eyes were red and the skin on my lips was flaking off. 'What did you do?' was ringing in my head like painful tinnitus.

We don't talk nearly enough about what happens after a suicide attempt. I didn't know how to process what had happened. It felt like I had dropped a nuclear bomb into the foundation of my life and everyone around me was caught in the blast. People walked on eggshells around me. My mum held onto my medications for months after, and I let her because it made her feel safe. When I went on a walk unannounced, my dad circled the neighbourhood in his car to make sure I was okay.

I felt traumatized by my near-death experience and intensely guilty for it. It took me years to talk about it in therapy, and even longer before I could accept that what happened was an actual trauma. Only then could I start to forgive myself, letting go of all the shame I had clung onto for so long.

I never for a moment could have imagined that this experience would be one I'd go through, but with help I got better.

This is why I believe it is so important that we acknowledge suicide can touch any of our lives. Talking about it doesn't invite it, but it can mean that we and our loved ones get the help we need. I still get the occasional suicidal ideation or odd thought during emotionally intense periods, but several things have helped me through those moments. Grounding and self-soothing techniques, which we get into more from page 116, have been helpful. Reminding myself that my feelings aren't permanent, and thinking about all the things I would have missed if I'd been 'successful' that first attempt, helps put things into perspective. I think a big part of suicide prevention is consciously adding moments of joy and things to look forward to in our everyday lives, as well as managing stress.

AFTER AN ATTEMPT

try to plan things for the upcoming weeks to look forward to - it can be small things like your favourite takeout or seeing a new movie

don't isolate! get connected with people and maintain your relationships

take time to process and try to be kind to yourself through these difficult feelings

reduce your daily stress as much as possible

identify the source of your suicidal thoughts, ask yourself:
- when did I first feel this way and what triggered it?
- what makes me feel better and what makes me feel worse?
- is there anything i could do, or get help to do, to feel more at peace in my life?

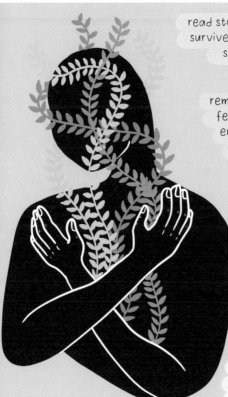

read stories about people who survived and recovered from suicidal thoughts

remember that it's normal to feel relief, disappointment, embarrassment or anger following an attempt

prioritize your healing by engaging in self-care and focusing on your recovery

join a support group in person or online

create a 'coping kit' with things that make you feel comforted, like a childhood stuffed animal, old photographs, favourite sweet treat, etc.

talk about your attempt with a professional or someone you trust

make an emergency plan for the future - who to call, what coping tools to use, a safe place to go, etc.

enrich your life by learning something new, like trying a new hobby or joining a class

IF YOU FEEL SUICIDAL

call emergency services if you need help right away

sit down and write out your feelings, you can write about things you love or things you'd like to do one day, or write a letter to your older self

step outside and feel the sun or wind on your skin and try to feel connected to the world around you

make yourself something delicious to eat and drink, and make yourself more comfortable

tell someone how you're feeling: a family member, a friend, or a suicide hotline, for example

steady your breathing and focus on your senses to ground your thoughts

try a self-harm coping technique, like tearing something apart or taking a cold shower

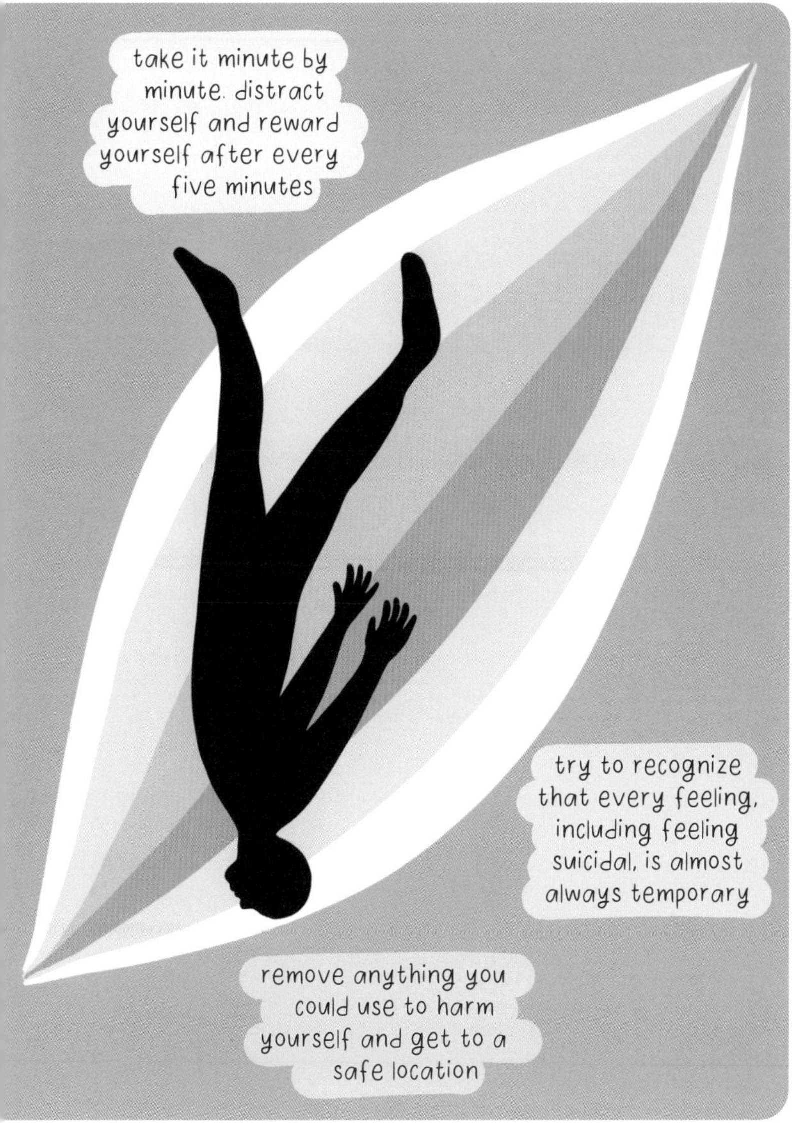
take it minute by minute. distract yourself and reward yourself after every five minutes
try to recognize that every feeling, including feeling suicidal, is almost always temporary
remove anything you could use to harm yourself and get to a safe location

Trauma lives in the body

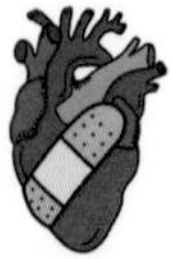

The following section describes my experiences of sexual assault and witnessing an accident. I've included these stories because they're an important part of my own mental health experiences, but if you don't want to read about them right now, then skip to page 56.

Trauma is more common than you might think. Though we might usually equate a traumatic event to things like surviving war or natural disaster, things like going through a divorce, a physical injury, the sudden loss of a loved one, or witnessing domestic violence as a child are also examples of traumatic events. Childhood trauma can affect us as adults: there are screening tests for what's called Adverse Childhood Experiences. People who have a high ACE score are more likely to struggle with things like substance abuse, chronic depression, toxic stress, and much more. Going through a traumatic event heightens the risk of mental health problems, so it's very important to look back on our lives and ask ourselves if we have any unhealed trauma that might be affecting us today.

My late teens were a blur because of trauma. At seventeen I had been in therapy for a couple of years, and felt quite stable and empowered. My recovery was put to the test when I survived a sexual assault, without even realizing it was assault at first, an experience I'm sure many people can relate to. It was simply something that happened while I was away at a music festival, and then my brain, in attempt to protect me, put it away deep below my conscious thoughts. That hazy night, then a

UNHEALED TRAUMA
CAN LOOK LIKE

low sense of
self-worth

keeping busy to
avoid confronting
the trauma

codependency
in relationships

tolerating abusive
or disrespectful
behaviour

fear of being
abandoned

resisting positive
change

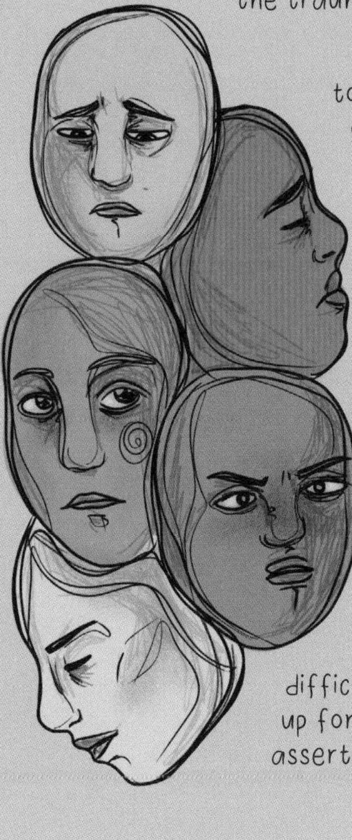

putting your
needs aside for
other people

always fearing
what might
happen next

craving
external
validation

difficulty standing
up for yourself and
asserting boundaries

an innate
feeling of
shame

not being able
to tolerate
conflict

YOUR TRAUMA IS VALID EVEN IF ...

it happened a long time ago

you never told anyone

you cant remember all of it

you didn't realize it was traumatic until later on

people didn't believe you

your life wasn't threatened

you are feeling better now

you know of people who have been through 'worse'

it didn't develop into PTSD

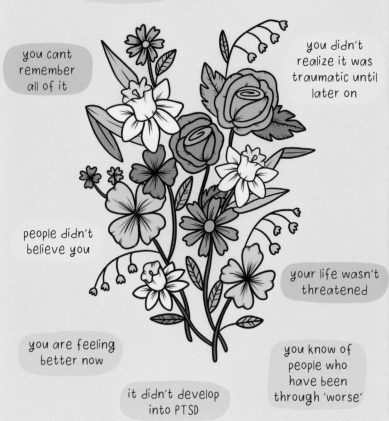

retraumatizing visit to the youth clinic, and life went on. It didn't come up until my first boyfriend said to me, 'You know you don't have to say yes to sex if you're not feeling like it, right?' In the safety of that moment my brain finally understood what had happened, and how wrong it was. But still, back in the box it went, because of how unspeakable it felt.

Meanwhile, the trauma of that night was taking its toll of my subconscious: I started to restrict my eating, as if I wanted to shrink away completely. The only thing that grew that year was my fearfulness around men.

The box I'd put that trauma away in stayed shut for a year, until the next domino dropped, when I witnessed a fatal road accident while road-tripping in America. This traumatic memory is starkly different from my previous one; the assault was all fuzzy and dreamlike, while this memory is clear as day, almost like I could step inside it and experience it all over again.

We had stopped for a cigarette break at sunset, and were interrupted by a loud boom nearby. Fearing it might be gunshots we got back in the car, but then we drove past it: a car ahead of us on the road, laying on its side, the wheels facing us. My boyfriend reassured me as we passed it, 'See, ambulances are coming,' but I told him what I'd seen in the car, on the road. It was too late.

As we continued our drive, every time I closed my eyes I could see the accident in vivid detail. After that, long after the trip was over, I had nightmares about accidents every night, about blood and death and glass – I'd wake up exhausted. In cars, my hands and feet would get tingly and numb, and my heart would beat loudly in my throat and ears. Memories of my assault began to pop up in my head again, my battered subconscious no longer able to keep it in a box, and I felt scared and on edge constantly.

Months later, I was assigned a new therapist, and shortly after, I was diagnosed with post-traumatic stress disorder (PTSD).

I did a lot of work to help myself heal, with what few skills I had.

I had done some cognitive behavioural therapy, which for me meant facing my social fears to defeat my social anxiety disorder. The only way to stop being scared is to face whatever scares you, so I knew I needed to do just that.

It scared me to be in cars, so I kept saying yes to being driven around by friends and family. It scared me to be in the presence of men, so I tried to get to know my boyfriend's friends better, and sometimes I'd ask a male stranger for directions or the time.

I wrote about my traumas, I filled pages and pages with everything I could remember. I wrote them in order, I wrote lists of what I was thinking during the experiences, I wrote them as poetry or in rhyming singsong, I wrote angry letters to my assaulter and crumpled them up. When I was home alone I would describe the experiences out loud from start to finish, again and again.

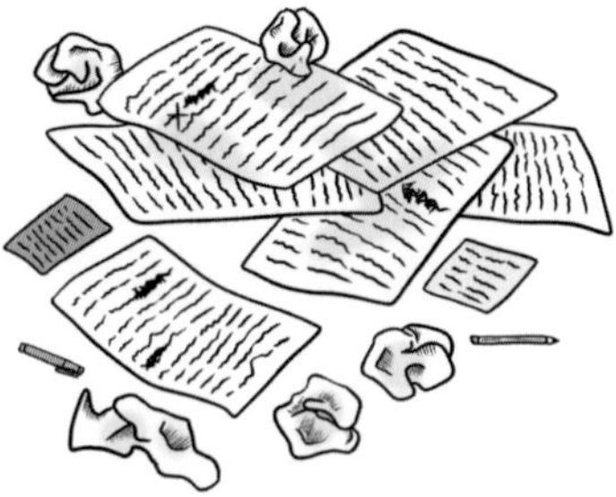

A lot of trauma therapy focuses on processing the trauma through remembering it again and again until it doesn't feel as intense. A trauma memory isn't like a normal memory; a trauma memory is disorganized, and fragmented. We don't remember trauma memories like we remember our more mundane memories – we relive them. Trauma work helps us assimilate and integrate those memories, giving them a start, a middle, and an end – to help our nervous system remember 'that was then, this is now', and in this now I am safe.

As I was working on healing my traumas, a lot of other stuff popped up – small traumas that I had forgotten about, or experiences that I didn't even realize were traumatic. Like being bullied at school as a child. Or having chronic migraines and struggling to find ways to cope with the intense pain of them. Or having a suicidal friend and being her only support at the age of twelve. All the things my childhood self had gone through were still somewhere inside, grating and hurting, appearing as random pains and aches and tension.

Trauma is so powerful, it is thought it can alter our genes and be passed down to our children; this is what's called 'intergenerational trauma'. It is not to be underestimated.

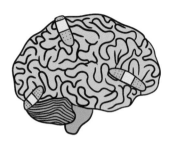

I kept journaling, talking with my partner and therapist, doing my fear-facing routines and collecting ways to cope. I avoided certain triggers like assault in movies by using websites like unconsentingmedia.org or doesthedogdie.com. I was patient with myself. After seven years of this, I don't think I would qualify for a diagnosis of PTSD any longer. The trauma memories still hurt, but they do not paralyze me. I'm not ruled by fear anymore. I think I would like to go to a festival with my friends again someday, and maybe even try to get my driving license, too.

If you are burdened by unresolved trauma, there are many ways to help yourself. Sometimes the things that make you feel better can be things you wouldn't expect. There are many things I've found useful and already mentioned but the main ones I'd suggest are:

- **Therapies**, such as EMDR (eye movement desensitization and reprocessing), neurofeedback and trauma-informed expressive arts therapy, are widely used to help process trauma.
- **Restorative yoga** is known to help your nervous system recover from trauma.
- **Breathwork**, such as taking slow purposeful breaths, helps the parasympathetic nervous system ('the rest and digest' system that helps us release tension) activate.

- **Reading forums** about trauma, as well as **books**, and **listening to podcasts**, helped me feel like there were communities of people who understood. Reading the book *The Body Keeps the Score* was especially validating and helpful in coming to terms with my traumas. Remember, it's okay to ask for help.

For me, the trauma of witnessing a fatal accident meant I had to ask for help, which then revealed past traumas I hadn't dealt with. Don't downplay your experiences – if you feel you've been through something traumatic, even if you feel you only 'might' need help, do speak to someone. Don't wait for trauma to build on trauma.

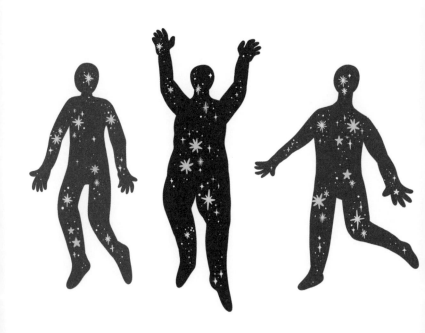

HEALING TRAUMA CAN LOOK LIKE

remembering that there's no right or wrong way to feel

trying to re-establish a sense of routine

reading books and seeking out information about trauma and options for coping

using movement to reconnect to your body, try rhythmic exercises that engage your limbs

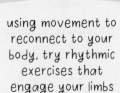

finding ways to healthily express feelings like anger, sadness and numbness

leaning on people you trust

listening to other survivors' stories and healing journeys

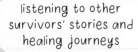

You are not broken

It's easy to feel alone when you're dealing with poor mental health. I thought I was especially ill, and that meant I needed to hide my inner turmoil because I figured it was deeply unrelatable and strange. But as I verbalized my feelings, I found much of what I was feeling and dealing with was shared by lots of people I know. Telling the truth about my pain, no matter how much shame I felt, opened doors to feel understood.

When we aren't properly taught to talk about hard feelings, or if we are not allowed to express them, we grow up ashamed or afraid of them. Sometimes we downplay the traumatic things we go through, and then things fester and linger. The first step of processing a feeling is acknowledging it. Reaching out for help is important, even if you're unsure if it's 'severe' enough, because if it hurts or bothers you, it's important to address it. It's easy to assume you're broken or that your mind is working against you when you don't have the tools to cope with feelings of inadequacy, stress, grief, or whatever difficulties life throws at you. But everyone can learn the art of feeling better if we give ourselves time, permission to ask for help or support, and patience and kindness with ourselves as we jump into the ebbs and flows of healing.

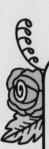

REMEMBER ...

We all have 'mental health'

•

Mental illness looks and feels
different for different people

•

Be aware of the warning
signs your mental health is
deteriorating

•

You can overcome your
traumas

•

Ask for help when you need it

Chapter 2

'WILL I EVER GET BETTER?' (YES!)

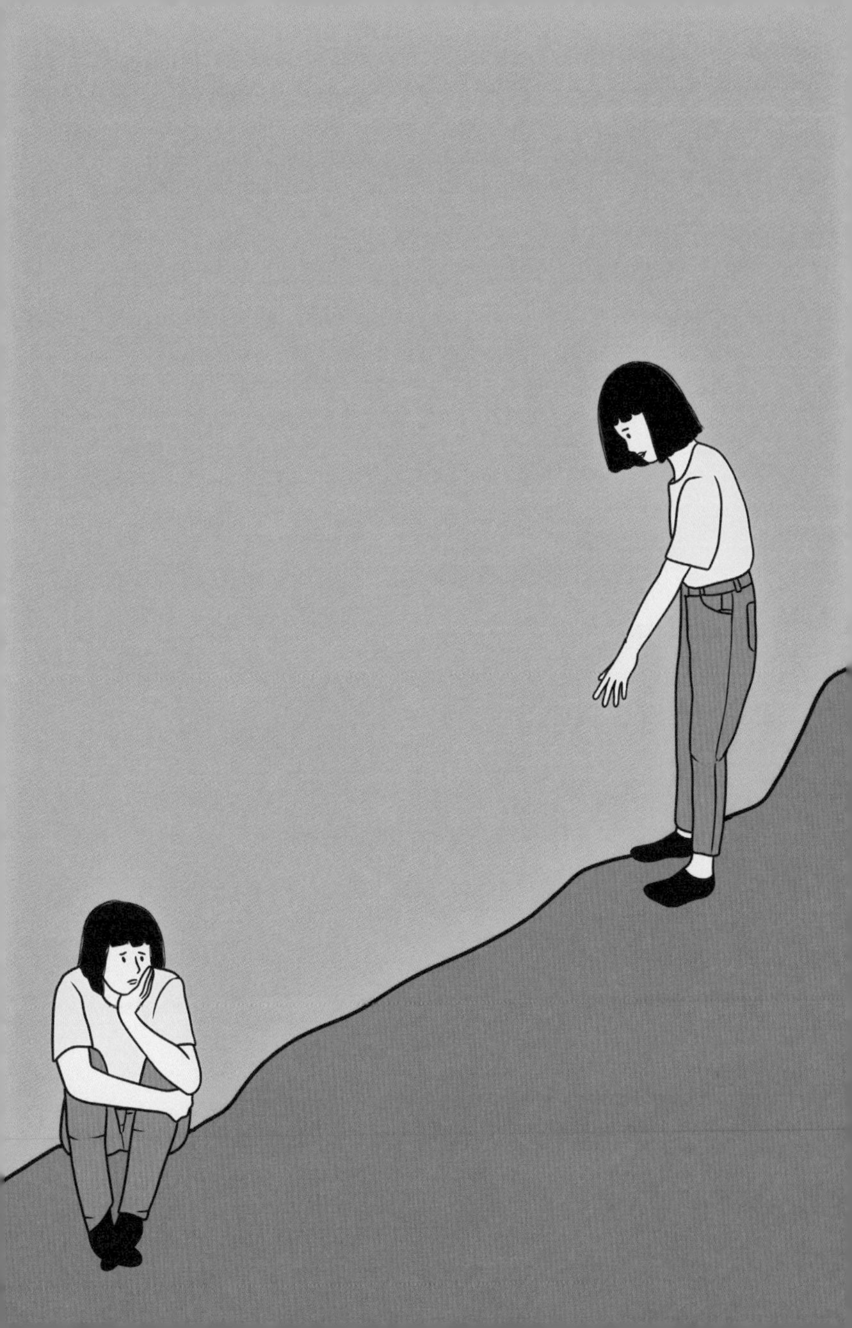

'I've tried everything and nothing works!'

At sixteen, as I was settling into regular therapy and started reading more intensely about psychology and the brain, particularly about my own diagnoses, I became obsessed with finding a cure. When someone had mental illness in

drinking water?
yoga?
being in nature?
art therapy?
prayer?
meditation?
Prozac?
exercise?
vitamins?
mindfulness?
aromatherapy?
cutting out sugar?
being on your phone less?
essential oils?
calling a hotline?
smiling more?
CBD?
keto?
thinking positively?
deep breathing?
CBT?

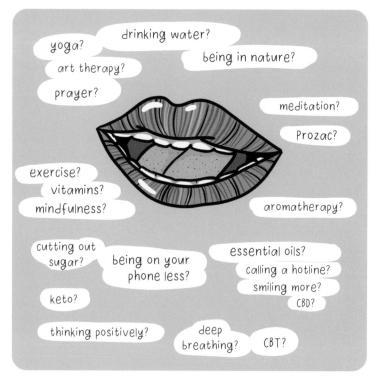

pop-culture media (and the character wasn't a serial killer) they'd hit rock bottom and then have a eureka moment in therapy that changed everything, and perhaps there was a getting better montage and – poof! They were cured right before the end credits. I had hit what felt like rock bottom, so where was my great eureka moment?

I tried everything suggested to me. Talk therapy, occupational therapy, cognitive behavioural therapy, group therapy. Antidepressants, sleeping medications, antipsychotics, mood stabilizers. To my horror, those things didn't instantly cure me, and all the emotional work of digging around in my brain felt like walking through a field of landmines. I couldn't tell if I was getting better or worse. It seemed like it was getting worse, because therapists kept finding more diagnoses.

That's when I discovered online wellness communities; influencers promoting detoxes, healthy eating and exercise as a way to become mentally well; positivity quotes like 'the difference between a good day and a bad day is your attitude'; and a well-known picture of a forest and below, a bunch of pills, with the caption, 'This is antidepressants, this is shit'. My impressionable young mind started questioning psychiatry – were my meds really just shit? Am I depressed because my attitude isn't optimistic enough, or because I lacked faith in a higher power? Have I not been outside enough, should I forego my medications and opt for the all-natural route?

Essential oils and vitamins and inspirational quotes did seem a lot easier than the intensive therapy that challenged my anxieties and made me feel extremely vulnerable. I started dabbling in yoga, researched daily habits of billionaires and took multivitamins. But, what do you know, I didn't find my eureka moment, nor my cure.

My problem wasn't that I was doing the wrong things. It was that I had modelled my expectations of recovery in an unrealistic way. I figured it was like having the flu – you get sick and you treat it and then you're as good as new.

Mental health is a bit more complicated. I didn't see a good day as something to celebrate because I knew it would end. Honestly, I didn't really start to get better until I completely let go of the need to be completely cured, and began prioritizing ways to help myself feel better about daily life. What if I let go of the pressure to be completely rid of any neuroses or symptoms, and started celebrating whenever I made any improvement, big or small? Just feeling 20% better would be much better; what if I could get to 50% better? What if I accepted the reality of my situation – that mental health can get worse and get better many times in a person's lifetime – and give myself some grace? If I recover completely, that would be great, but if I don't, it doesn't make life any less worth living. Even if I live my entire life as a person with mental health problems, that's okay, as long as I treat and manage my symptoms. Recovery wasn't a race to the finish line, but a walk that gets easier the more steps I take.

Professional help and treatments were important, but I also needed simple and low-effort things to help me cope when I was by myself and felt exhausted. Most of the wellness culture rhetoric I left behind, because I realized it was trying to sell me stuff, but I'll admit some things helped. Moving your body, practicing positivity and mindfulness can all be incredibly powerful when searching for better health. Not every therapeutic exercise I learnt worked for me, so I focused on the things that did, but I gave everything a chance. And I allowed myself to practice self-help in ways I enjoyed. Even though some people might say healing crystals are nonsense, I give them room in my repertoire because they make me feel good, alongside my breathing exercises and anxiety medication. The more ways of feeling better we discover, the more chances we have to fill our days with them and make life more fabulous.

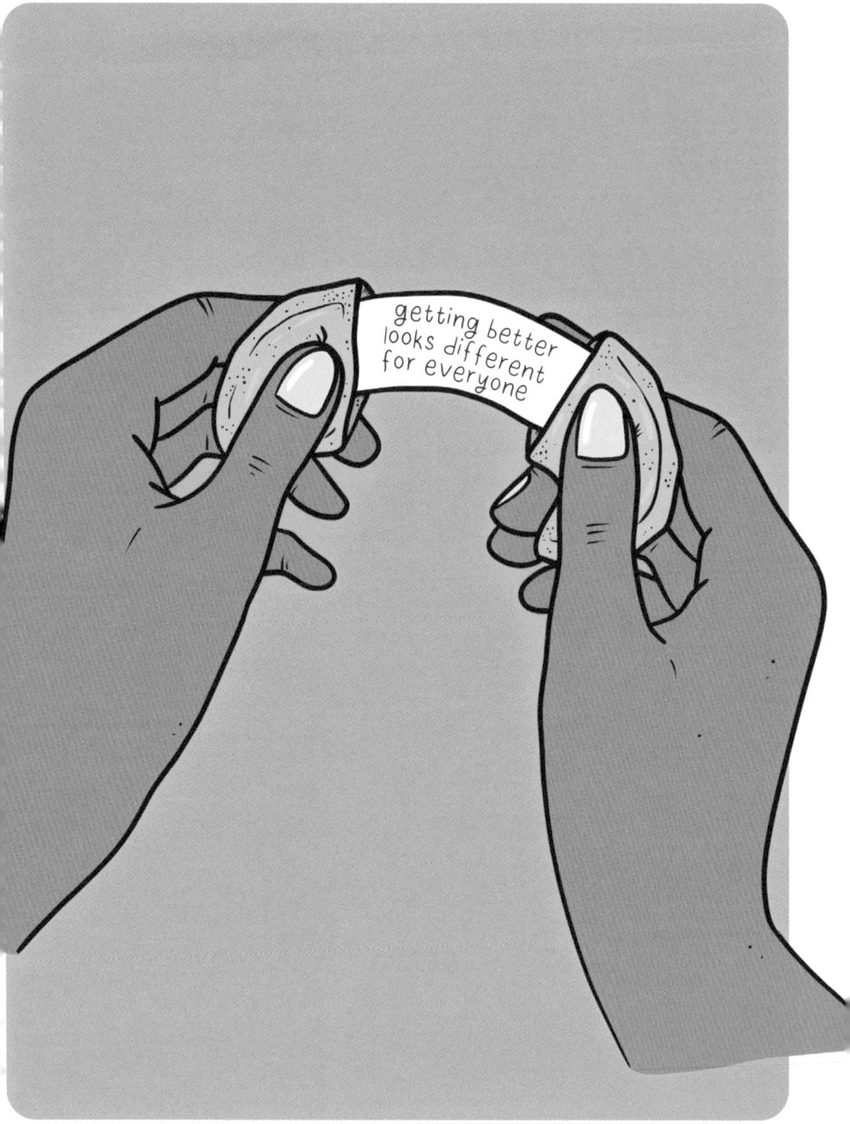
getting better
looks different
for everyone

Healing is possible

There's this feeling that followed me around for years. It started as a little seed of self-doubt when I was a kid and started school, it grew bigger and bigger as I moved through my teen years. A soreness, a stubborn ache that moved from my stomach to my heart to the tips of my fingers, like a painful ingrown nail or a kernel stuck in my throat, too deep to reach in and fish it out. I tried ignoring it, and when that didn't work, I tried drinking, smoking, sweating and eating it away. It worked for brief moments, but after a night out I came back to bed and was greeted by that familiar pain. A part of me knew it was something I should probably be alarmed by, and that it needed to be dealt with, but the other part of me was tired, and she did everything to avoid opening a psychological can of worms.

In high school I met my mentor, my art teacher Nadia. Us meeting was nothing short of cosmic; she had travelled her own path to healing, which gave her an amazing ability to turn the school's art studio into a safe space for her students. Nadia invited open conversations about mental health. Her office was always open for a cry-session if we were exhausted from life, and she asked us how we genuinely felt. She didn't allow the her curriculum to come before our mental health, she was so warm and caring. Once she invited me to come to trauma-informed yoga; another time she

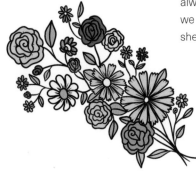

brought in a woman who held guided meditation with us because she knew school was a lot. She sometimes offered up stories of her own journey of healing, which helped inspire my own. Nadia helped me realize that there is no healing without surrendering to vulnerability. When I left high school, I was ready to untangle and explore that pain within. When I allowed myself to dissect that unidentified pain, which happened when I consciously chose to sit with my feelings and let them be felt, instead of reaching for distractions, it became clear that it was a culmination of unresolved emotions from all the times I didn't know how to process my feelings. The more I dug, the more memories revealed themselves; it was painful. My subconscious mind had built a hefty shield around my traumas to protect me, and it was up to my conscious mind to dissemble it.

I visualized my younger self in the moments she was hurting. I told her all the things she didn't get to hear but so desperately needed to hear. I cried for her until I was swollen and red-faced. Closing my eyes, I imagined cradling her in my arms and squeezing out her hurt from every microscopic pore. I wrote scathing letters to my schoolyard bullies detailing my reactions to their actions, I wrote odes to lost friendships. Lists of everything bad that ever happened, over and over again until I had processed every little detail. When all the notes had piled up on my desk and my brain was quiet, I ripped them all into tiny pieces and stuffed them in the bin. Emotional pain revealed itself physically as headaches, stiffness and tension in my body, so I stretched and moved. When confronted with hurt, I shook my body vigorously, like something feral, as if infested with ants, until I was exhausted and gasping for air. When I was stressed, 'shaking it out' was my go-to. I vowed to feel; to cry when I felt sad, to express my anger when it crept up, to remind myself that I am ready to face difficult feelings – that my feelings are telling me things that I must examine. To never again let it build up until it overflows and explodes.

HEALING CAN LOOK LIKE

learning to dwell a little less and dream a little more

giving space for difficult feelings

welcoming support and asking for help without self-judgement

being able to do things outside of your comfort zone

being able to set, enforce and communicate your boundaries

feeling comfortable expressing your needs, feelings and opinions

feeling safe within yourself and in your relationships with others

feeling more in control of yourself and your reactions

not automatically blaming and shaming yourself when things go wrong

managing your emotions and letting them guide you towards self-improvement

having more positive and calm thoughts

being less fixated on things you can't change and focusing more on things you can change

dealing better with disappointment and setbacks

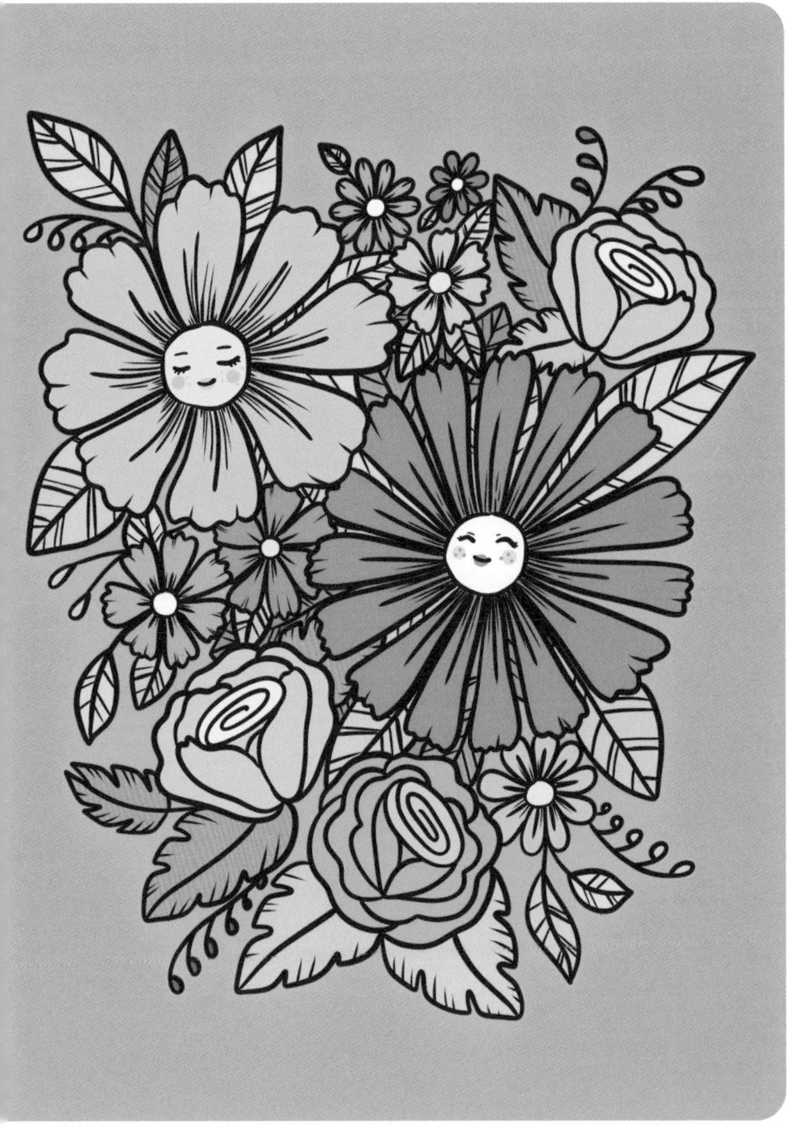

When facing emotional pain, or when you find yourself repeating unhelpful habits or ruminating on the same negative thoughts, ask yourself, what is this telling you? What do you need to do so you can heal? What needs to be added to the story before you can finish that chapter? Healing is a process that spans our entire lives, and during difficult times, we need to honour ourselves by prioritizing it. Be patient, because healing happens moment by moment, a day at a time.

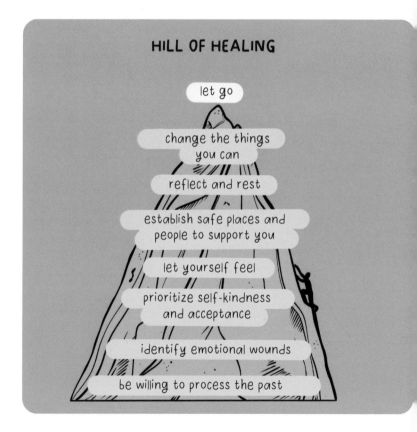

HILL OF HEALING

let go

change the things you can

reflect and rest

establish safe places and people to support you

let yourself feel

prioritize self-kindness and acceptance

identify emotional wounds

be willing to process the past

Optimism is a life raft

Do you feel helpless against your own thoughts sometimes? Do you wonder if other people's minds are also full of harsh self-criticism?

In my mid-teens, at the start of my mental health journey, people would relentlessly remind me of the 'power of positivity', much to my annoyance. I detested being told to try to be more optimistic, as if it was an easy thing for me to do while watching my entire life fall apart. What was there to be positive about when waking up in the mornings felt like the start of another nightmare? It felt impossible that it might help, because I'd definitely be faking it.

This attitude persisted until I learned more about neuroscience and neuroplasticity (the brain's ability to change and adapt its function and structure), and discovered that our thoughts become our reality. Repeated negative thought patterns, as they create pathways in the brain that are used so often, become our beliefs, and those beliefs go on to influence our view on the world and ourselves, as well as our behaviour. To some extent, the quality of our thoughts becomes the quality of our lives. I had become trapped in a vicious cycle of negative thinking, and with this new-found realisation, I was desperate to claw my way out.

It turns out that the positivity I hated so much was 'toxic positivity', the kind of false reassurance some people give when they'd rather dismiss your negative emotions because they're unequipped to deal with it. Toxic positivity forces you to push aside negative emotions, while genuine optimism acknowledges the negative feelings, but encourages you to get through them.

I like to imagine optimism as a muscle in my body; it needs regular exercise to become stronger. Positive affirmations sounded disingenuous to me because I had been telling myself negative affirmations all my life. My head was a loop of 'not good enough', 'not worthy', 'I will fail', 'bad things always happen to me'. My first affirmation was a simple, 'Everything's gonna be okay'. I repeated it as soon as I felt anxious, or embarrassed, or sad. I'd say it out loud to myself before bed, in the mornings as I greeted my reflection, as a mumble on the bus. For weeks and weeks the sentence lived in my head as a mantra. And then, it stopped sounding like a lie – I had started to believe it. I had built a bit of trust in myself, and I could feel a shift in my mindset. I was looking for positive truths to challenge negative beliefs. Those negative thoughts didn't disappear, but it was easier to distance myself from them. I told myself that the negative thoughts were unfounded self-criticism and that the positive thoughts were my kinder self, cheering me on.

It's hard to start to shift your mindset when you feel like you have to force it at first. You might feel silly or disingenuous as you first try out affirmations and positive self-talk. When I started I kept thinking, 'What's the point of these affirmations if I'm just lying to myself, and if I'm aware I'm lying?' This is a common first hurdle when starting out, and it's completely understandable. Building confidence isn't a quick-fix, it's a gradual process like almost everything else. A good starting out affirmation, one that deals with the awkwardness of it all, could simply be: 'There is a part of me that thinks I don't deserve to be confident or kind to myself, but I'm showing myself that I'm worth it by reminding myself of my value.' Or: 'This makes me feel stupid but it's just because I have to practice it every day, and there's nothing stupid about being nice to myself.'

Learning to be okay with feeling awkward is part of processing uncomfortable emotions; we can do things that makes us feel silly without judging ourselves.

TOXIC POSITIVITY

being negative won't help you

good vibes only!

you'll get over it

other people have it a lot worse

smile, crying won't help you

just stay positive

GENUINE OPTIMISM

it's important to let ourselves feel our feelings

i love you through all your emotional states

i believe you can get through this, and I'm here to help

you're not alone in this

everyone needs a good cry now and then. can i get you a tissue or give you a hug?

things are tough right now, do you want to talk about it, or do something more lighthearted?

Developing a growth mindset

The term 'growth mindset' was coined by Carol Dweck in the mid-2000s. People with growth mindsets believe that we can evolve and improve our skills if we put in effort and nurture ourselves.

Having a fixed mindset, on the other hand, means that one believes their talents and skills are static, that we are limited by the things

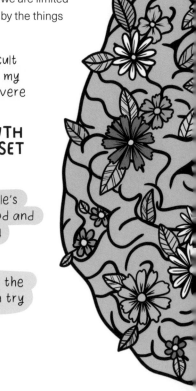

i can do difficult things if i try my best and persevere

i don't have to be the best at something for it to be meaningful

GROWTH MINDSET

other people's success is good and inspiring

failure can help me learn

If i don't get it the first time, i can try again

i can learn to do anything i want

that challenge us. People with fixed mindsets can't believe they will succeed or improve at doing hard things. It ties into learned helplessness; the more convinced we are that we cannot escape our current situation, the more likely we are to give up trying to break free, because of our perceived lack of control. We become stuck; even when we are able to escape, we don't, because we don't believe in our own abilities anymore.

A growth mindset can help us remember that failure doesn't define us, it only informs us of where we are in our unique journey, and serves as an invitation to persevere. Challenges are welcomed because, whether we succeed or not, we can praise ourselves for the effort and try again without letting failure define us negatively.

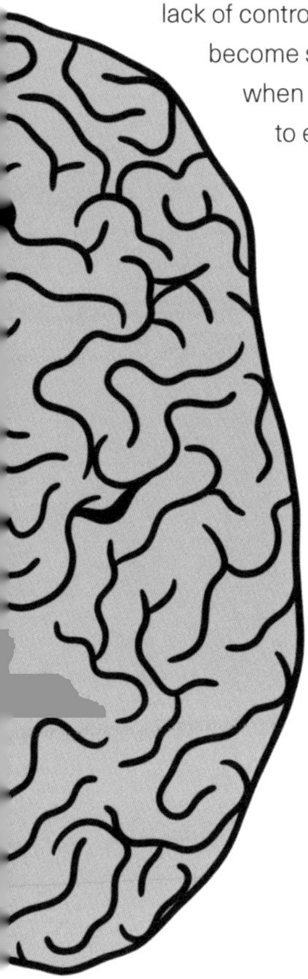

i'm not good enough to do this

FIXED MINDSET

failure shows that i'm incapable of achieving what i want

other people's success is a proof of my failure

if i'm not excelling, it's not worth it

my abilities are fixed

if i can't do it now, i will never be able to

As a child, I had a natural growth mindset: I was curious and eager to try, without feeling pressured to 'succeed'. I learned by play and creative pursuits, and felt inspired by the talents of others. But as I grew and began to enter the 'real world', I started believing that effort could only be rewarded if it lead to success. It wasn't fun to explore my abilities or try new things – if I wasn't immediately able to grasp something, I had failed, and in my eyes, failure felt unacceptable and shameful. All of this triggered negative thoughts about myself, creating those neural pathways, until I didn't believe I was capable of anything. A big theme of the affirmations I started revolved around redefining what success meant to me, and trying to get back to that natural growth mindset from childhood.

what's the point of trying if you're just going to fail anyway?

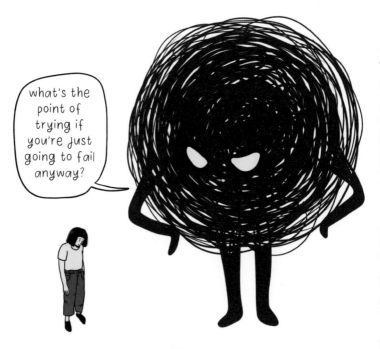

Letting go of expectations

As you begin to challenge negative thoughts, you might notice the negative self-belief that they stem from.

As I challenged these negative thoughts, I kept discovering all these beliefs I didn't even know I held, ones that were deeply embedded and not at all supportive of my mental health – societal attitudes and expectations, as well as my own expectations of myself. As a young woman, I've spent my whole life being conditioned to be constantly aware of my imperfections, to be self-sacrificing, nurturing, accommodating, polite. The people who are praised, adored and popular in our world are those who succeed, those who are beautiful, charismatic, and effortlessly talented, whose lives seem easy and rich in opportunity.

As a child I understood life as a series of milestones, on a set timeline. You get good grades, a sensible degree, a respectable job, you get married and pay off a mortgage and have children and maybe a golden retriever, and then you're all set.

I was taught that to achieve happiness I had to be a good kid, a good student, a good worker, a productive member of society.

When I left school I applied for jobs working with special educational needs students, because I didn't get help with my learning disabilities in school, and I wanted to help kids who struggled in similar ways to me. But the intense workload didn't mix well with my mental health, no matter how much I cared for my students. So how could I be good if I flunked out of high school and kept losing all my jobs and couldn't bring myself to jump in the shower during bouts of depression?

Living up to societal expectations felt like chasing a moving target, always just out of reach.

After I lost my last job, I finally asked myself: who am I doing all this for? Because the chase certainly wasn't making me happy. Expectations are arbitrary in a world as vast as ours. Other people's expectations of you are their problem, not yours. Relinquishing the beliefs I had about what makes a person good or worthy was the ultimate unlearning.

As much as I love service-oriented work and am drawn to helping others, those environments don't work for me, and I need to help myself before I can help others. My love for art has been lifelong, and I always dreamt of being a professional artist, so I decided to put my all into commissions and odd illustration jobs – and after a while all those little incomes became a liveable wage. Not as much as at my previous jobs, but enough

to get by. Being my own boss and dealing with the uncertainty of freelancing is overwhelming sometimes, but forging my own way was necessary for my health.

It was uncomfortable to realize that I valued approval and validation more than I valued my authentic self, but nothing was as beneficial as challenging that belief. It didn't matter if certain people approved of my decisions, because I wasn't choosing for them, but for me.

It's important to question the things we already think we know, especially beliefs about what makes us good or 'enough'. A lot of us walk around carrying beliefs and ideas that don't serve us, that take away our joy. So I invite you to take this opportunity to examine your beliefs and thoughts about yourself: are they kind or are they harsh?

THINGS I AM
UNLEARNING

making myself
smaller to fit into
social situations

ignoring my own
boundaries to
please other people

sacrificing my
voice or beliefs to
avoid conflict

pretending that
i'm fine instead of
asking for support

believing my
self-worth
depends on my
productivity

not celebrating my
accomplishments
because they're
'small'

societal standards
of beauty, and
diet-culture
mentality

distracting from
hard feelings
instead of
processing them

seeking external
validation over
self-assurance

UNLEARNING STATEMENTS

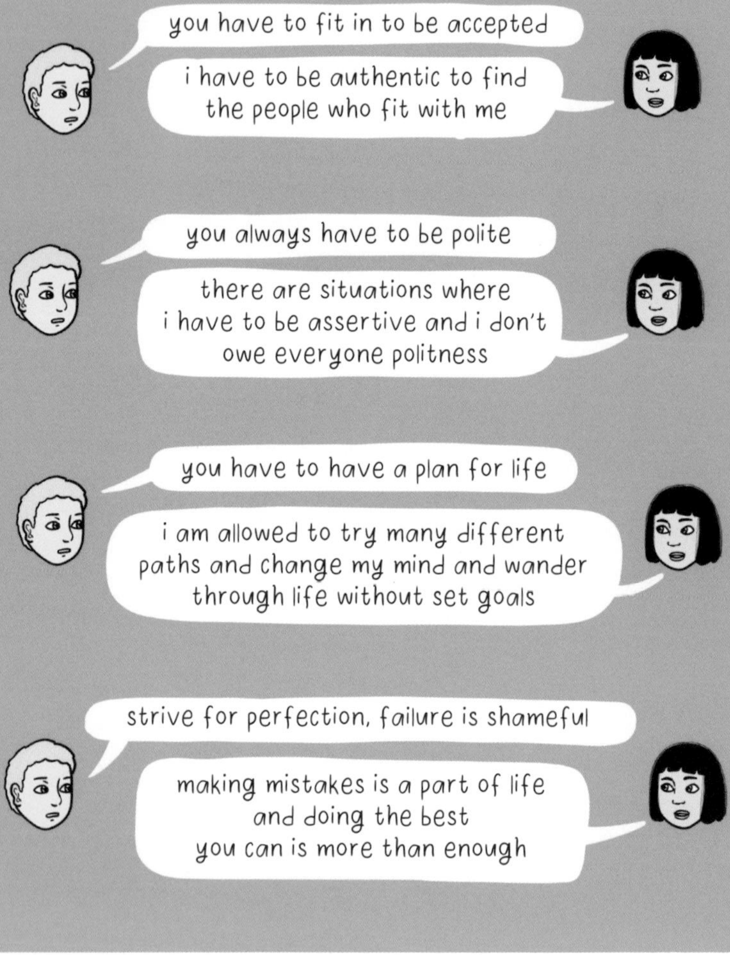
you have to fit in to be accepted
i have to be authentic to find the people who fit with me
you always have to be polite
there are situations where i have to be assertive and i don't owe everyone politness
you have to have a plan for life
i am allowed to try many different paths and change my mind and wander through life without set goals
strive for perfection, failure is shameful
making mistakes is a part of life and doing the best you can is more than enough

How you look and why it doesn't matter

Body image issues can be the catalyst for an array of mental health problems. Dissatisfaction with our physical appearance can take a huge toll on our self-esteem; it's a risk factor for psychological distress and unhealthy behaviours.

My issues with my body were planted like seeds throughout my adolescence – by adults who discussed diets and their own dissatisfaction with themselves in my presence, by classmates who compared and commented in the changing rooms at school. Little by little I noticed just how much importance is placed on the physical. Our body image does not form in isolation and we are not born with body insecurity.

It is something we learn from the media and attitudes that surround us every day, and the pressure to conform to an ideal can feel inescapable.

As a child I assumed I would grow out of my awkward looks and blossom into a beautiful woman like the ones I saw in movies, but I never grew out of an A-cup and my body never developed into an hourglass shape. Instead, I grew taller than the girls in my class, broad-shouldered and pear-shaped.

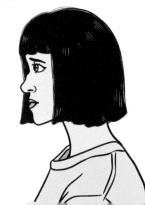

I started picking apart everything about myself, and my search history turned into a long list of desperate queries like, 'How to get thicker hair', 'How to get rid of hip dips', 'What do normal labia look like' and 'Why do my boobs point sideways'. My biggest insecurity was my nose. My family all have a nose with a bump, and mine is the most prominent of them all. I felt this ruined my looks – there it is, sitting right in the centre of my face, unable to be hidden. I decided that plastic surgery was the only option for what I deemed a facial deformity, and I would daydream of surgery and showing off my new 'normal' nose.

Around the same time, the idea of body positivity exploded on social media. As a social movement, the aim of body positivity is to promote the acceptance of all bodies, and to challenge beauty standards as an unwelcome social construct.

It was inspiring to me and I decided that I wanted in on it – I was desperately craving peace with myself. But no matter how assertively I told myself my nose was beautiful just the way it is, it felt like a ludicrous lie every time. How could it be beautiful when the only time I saw my nose represented was as the 'before picture' on a plastic surgery website? It felt unrealistic to love my body when I'd compare myself to what I saw on every screen or magazine.

After giving up any hope of coming to terms with myself, I stumbled upon the term 'body neutrality', and it changed my life. Body neutrality isn't about loving the way we look no matter what, but instead takes the focus off of the way we look entirely. It reminds us that we are multifaceted beings and that our physical appearance is the least important thing about us. This resonated with me when I thought about what I admire in the people I love, like their humour, interests, our conversations, their kindness – not the way they look.

I started to challenge why it was so important for me to fit into the ideal, how beauty is a form of currency in our society, and how classist our standards of beauty are.

The more deeply I thought about what I understood as

physical attractiveness, especially the beauty standards that female-presenting/identifying people face, the more dehumanizing I found it. Like, am I not allowed to feel good in a body that grows hair, has spots and scars, and will one day wrinkle and sag? Why must I shrink and pluck and cover the natural texture of my skin? I started purposefully leaving my armpits unshaven, despite the looks I'd get in public. I left my pimples uncovered, I pierced my nose with golden hoops even though it drew attention to it, I started only doing things with my body that I wanted, that made me feel happy: decisions that weren't influenced by the ideal, but by my own comfort. I stopped putting on makeup to do a quick grocery run, and I grew more accustomed to my face at is it, bare and imperfect. I moved my body because it felt good, not to get toned or look more fit.

I don't exist to be easy on the eyes. My time is better spent learning new things, working on my development and healthy habits, not spending my every waking moment hyper-fixated on how I look through the eyes of others. I don't owe anyone a perfectly straight nose, and I don't need to measure up to beauty standards, because they don't matter. I don't want to look back at my life when I'm old and regret how long I wasted worrying about the way I look.

As I started to consciously push aside thoughts about my appearance, the less I felt the need to be beautiful, and the easier it was to appreciate myself for who I am. Starting with body positivity felt like

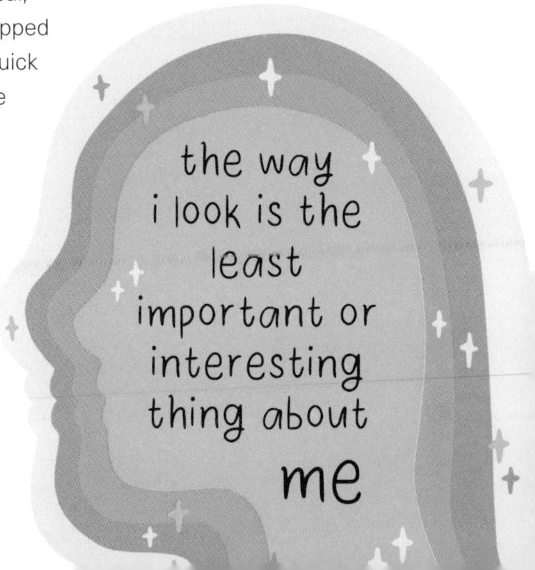
the way
i look is the
least
important or
interesting
thing about
me

biting off more than I could chew, while body neutrality was a much easier first step to free myself from desperately adhering to the standards of beauty. You can't lose if you decide that you're not playing the vanity game anymore, and I was done with it.

If you're struggling with your body image, know that it's possible to improve the way you feel about yourself. Think of someone in your life who you love. If you were to write a list of why you love them, ask yourself, is the way they look on that list? Is it higher up than how they make you feel, the values they have? More important than your conversations together, their humour or compassion or kindness? Probably not, right?

Do you find little flaws and imperfections endearing on other people but not yourself? Would you call yourself ugly if your younger self was listening? Would you ever say to others what you think about yourself, or are you only bothered by imperfection when it's you? What would happen if you started to

compliment yourself, and comfort yourself, like you can do to others?

Extreme body image issues can feel impossible to break out of, but we really are the architects of our thoughts. A first step to feeling more comfortable in our bodies is diverting our focus to other things when we have negative thoughts about how we look. It can help our brains realize that the aesthetic state of our bodies aren't to be prioritized over everything else. If you notice that you are missing out on experiences, hyper-fixating on 'flaws' to the point that it rules your life, or constantly hiding or checking your 'flaws', it might be time to reach out to someone you trust. Doing things to take care of your body in healthy ways, such as with proper nutrition and fun, gentle exercises, practicing mindfulness, or finding a support group online or in your area can all help rebuild your relationship with your body. But if you find you can no longer engage in eating well and exercising sensibly without it becoming extreme, you should speak to someone you trust, like your doctor, a teacher, a parent or a friend.

Make friends with yourself again

You are a part of your own social support system. As the only person in your head, your job is vital within your support system. Only you know what happens in your thoughts, and how you feel in each moment. Are you a friend to yourself?

As a young child, I was my own best friend. I didn't mind playing with my classmates, but if the game didn't interest me I would happily decline and wander off, completely content in my own company. That all changed as I grew older, when I was introduced to social hierarchies and my mental health problems began to reveal themselves. The tween years were quite brutal; it didn't take much to upset me, which made me an easy target. I entered school with high self-esteem and left with none. How could I like myself when other people didn't? I started seeing myself as the enemy, the saboteur of my own life, constantly fantasizing about ways to change drastically so I could be accepted by anyone and everyone. It wasn't comfortable to sit in solitude anymore, it felt suffocating. Time alone had become a scheduled appointment for self-criticism, to sit and pick apart my face and body and personality, scouring for flaws and things to fix.

The friends I did gain, I loved unconditionally. I loved them even in the moments they flaked or we argued. Being a friend came easy, like my purpose on earth was loving others; but saving some of that love for myself felt impossible. I didn't see a reason to.

I vividly remember the moment I started to treat myself as a friend again. My high school creative writing class had organized a poetry reading after school, and any student was welcome to take the stage. My immediate reaction was horror, and a barrage of thoughts to the tune of 'I could never do that, I have terrible stage fright, I'd embarrass myself, I'm not good enough'. My friend turned to me and told me she wasn't sure if she wanted to perform at the reading. Without a second thought, I responded: 'Of course you should do it, your poems are so good! I know just the one you should do.'

And that got me thinking – why was it so easy to lift her up, but not myself? I decided I would do the reading too if I could gather up the courage.

The night of the poetry reading, I stood in the bathroom of the cafe, trembling and terrified, considering calling it quits and going home. But instead, I did something I had never done before. I looked my reflection in the eyes and said, 'You've got this. It will be okay.' When it was my turn on the stage, I stared at the fuzzy faces of my classmates and their families, my heart beating loudly in my ears. I started reading, my voice the only sound filling up the room. Then ... I had done it! The room erupted in applause and I was overcome by a sense of overwhelming pride. I felt incredible empowerment, and then a realization: imagine what else I could do if I encouraged myself? If I advocated for, supported and comforted myself? That evening I made a promise to treat myself as a friend once again. To save some of that love I give so freely to others, just for me.

correct negative self-talk and try not to say anything to yourself that you wouldn't say to a friend

advocate for your needs

celebrate your accomplishments and growth no matter how minor they may feel in the moment

HOW TO BE A FRIEND
TO YOURSELF

check in with
yourself. what are
your needs, wants,
fears, etc.?

give yourself praise
and compliments as
well as consolation
and compassion

be protective of your
energy and personal
boundaries

don't put
expectations on
yourself that you
wouldn't put on
others

encourage yourself
during difficult
times

make your health a
priority to yourself

be gentle with
yourself and allow
yourself to learn
from your mistakes

spend time alone
doing things that
you enjoy

focus on the things
that you like or
value about yourself

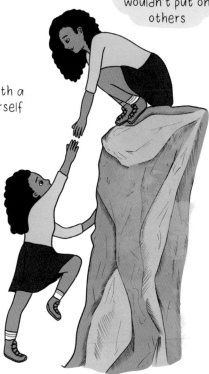

You are worth the work on yourself

It can feel demoralizing when you begin your journey of feeling better, because as we open ourselves up to assess and process inner feelings and external stresses, more and more points of hurt might pop up. Sometimes feeling better starts with letting yourself feel sad and hurt and angry about things you've repressed or distracted yourself from. It can feel like standing on the starting line of a marathon and seeing the long stretch of road ahead, thinking, 'I don't know if I can do this, I don't know if I'm strong enough, I don't feel safe in this moment.' But in the marathon of feeling better, it's okay not to run, it's okay to take small steps, to sit down and pause, to walk hand in hand with a friend. It's okay not to get to the finish line the first time, or the second or the third. But every time you try, you might notice yourself getting further and further, as your mind develops the muscles and stamina that you need to reach your destination.

Small accomplishments all add up to make noticeable change. Every self-destructive habit that we learn how to break is one step closer to feeling more at peace in your reality. Every time you challenge a negative thought you remind your inner critic that they aren't welcome to eat away at your happiness any longer. Every time you make a conscious effort to step in and be a friend to yourself, you teach yourself that you deserve love and care. Change doesn't happen overnight.

Mental health care is always worthwhile, no matter where you are in your personal journey. Much like learning any new skill, it takes daily practice, on your good days and bad days.

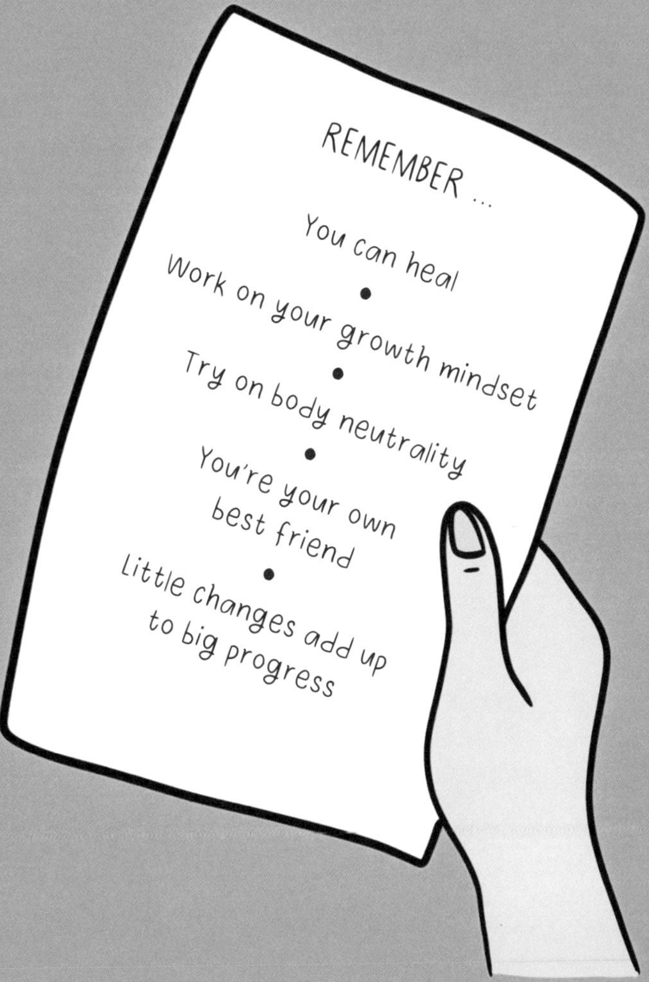
REMEMBER ...
You can heal
Work on your growth mindset
Try on body neutrality
You're your own best friend
Little changes add up to big progress

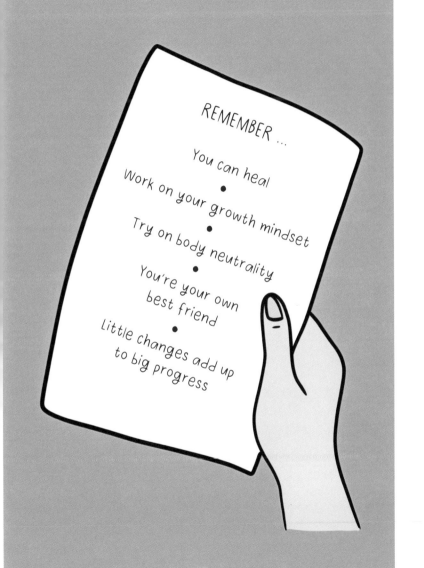

YOUR MENTAL HEALTH TOOLKIT

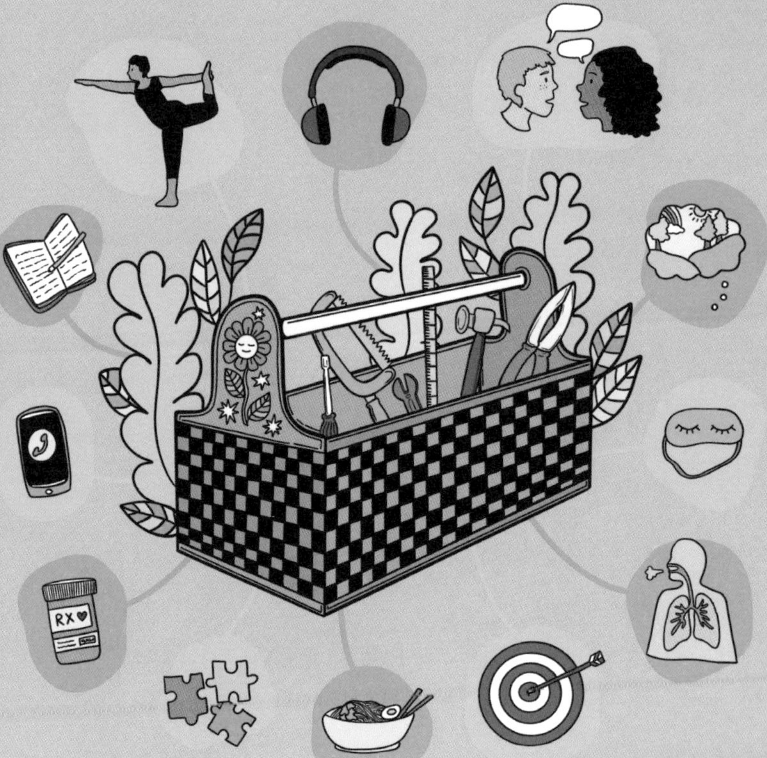
RX

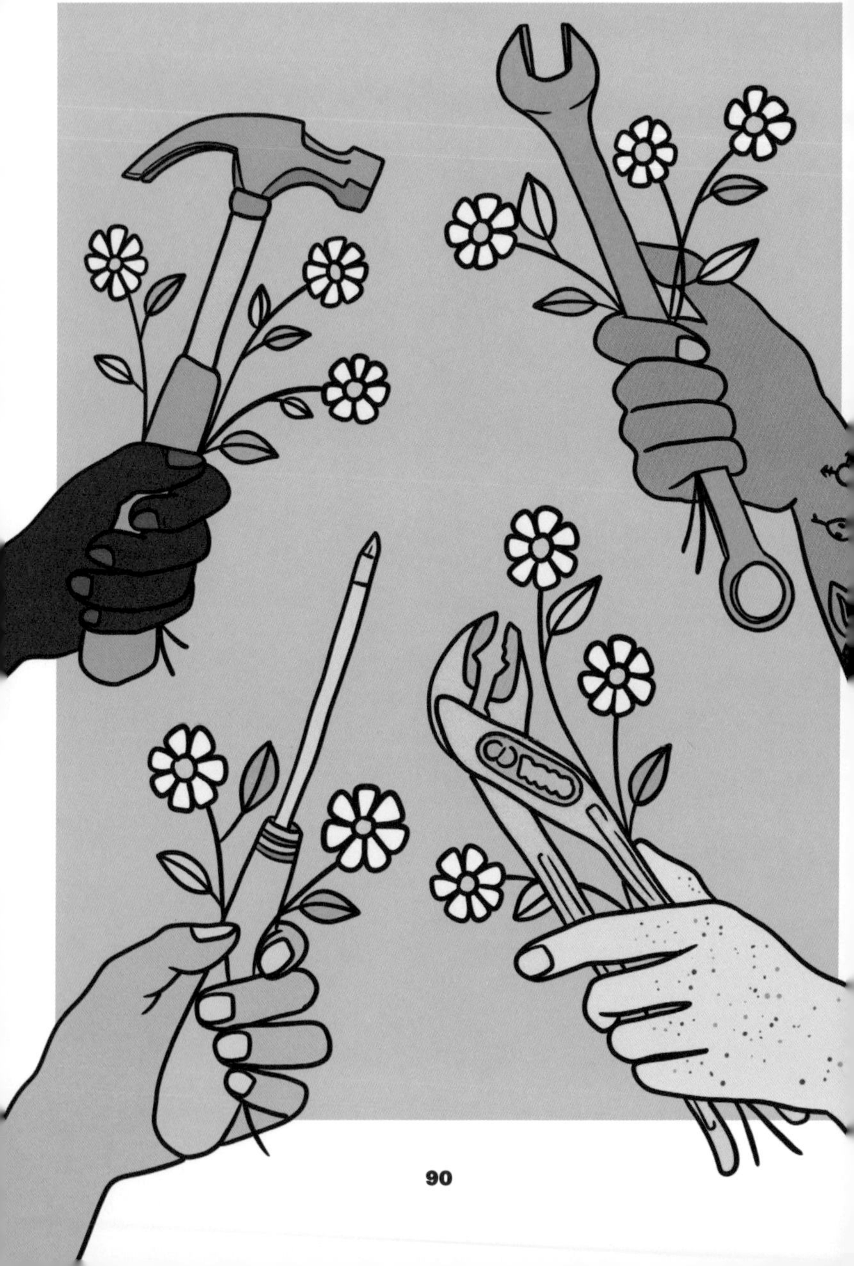

Tools for feeling better

To remember all the things that make me feel better, I started imagining them all put together in a toolbox. Much like the different tools that a carpenter uses to fix or build, I can take out an affirmation or a breathwork exercise as I need. I can dip into the self-care and coping skills that I've gathered over the years. The idea of having a mental space full of helpful tips and tricks can really help you to feel in control. Different problems require different solutions, so the easiest way to start building your own toolbox is to think about what feels wrong or overwhelming, and what things comfort you or help you practically.

In this chapter I invite you to peek into my toolbox and try a few things out for yourself. Take what you like, put aside what doesn't work for you. My toolbox has changed lot over the years; at the start of my own journey I tried medications to help me feel better, and found over time that I could come off them – but maybe one day I'll feel the need to try meds again. Our recoveries are fluid and the things that help during one period of time might not work later on, and vice versa. Give yourself grace and patience, and check in with yourself to see what your needs are in your current state.

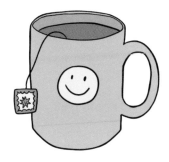

Self-compassion 101

There are times I wonder when the mean voice of self-judgment first popped into my head. Maybe it started as a subconscious echo of all the negative attitudes that are unavoidable in society, every

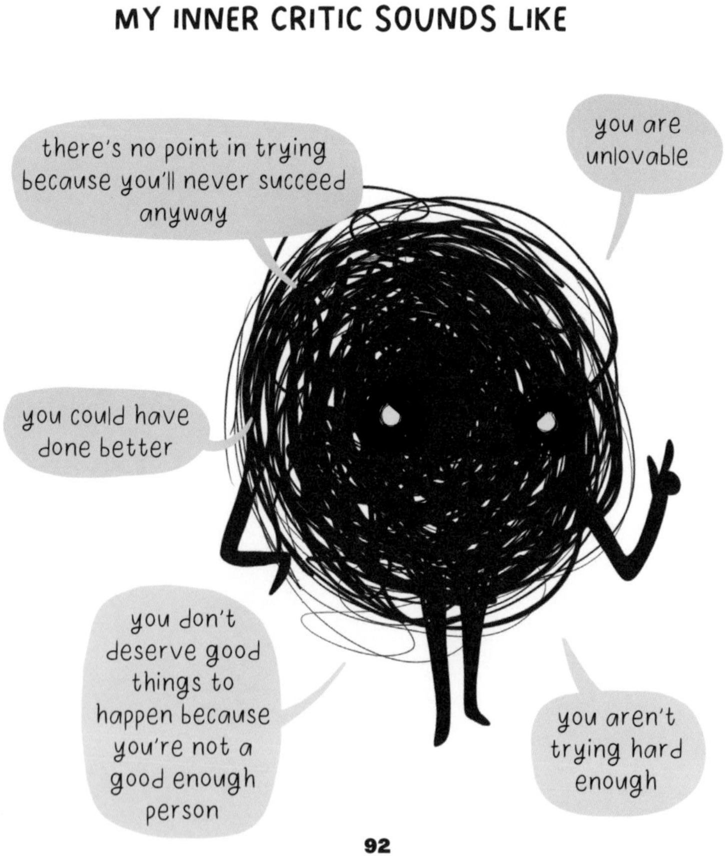
MY INNER CRITIC SOUNDS LIKE
there's no point in trying because you'll never succeed anyway
you are unlovable
you could have done better
you don't deserve good things to happen because you're not a good enough person
you aren't trying hard enough

expectation and norm I couldn't fulfil, all piling up and solidifying as an evil version of myself in my head, whose sole purpose was to tear me down. Every accomplishment was spoiled by that voice saying, 'Well, anyone could have done that, it's nothing special'. If I got a B on a difficult test, the voice would remind me that 'your friends all got As so you're still not good enough'.

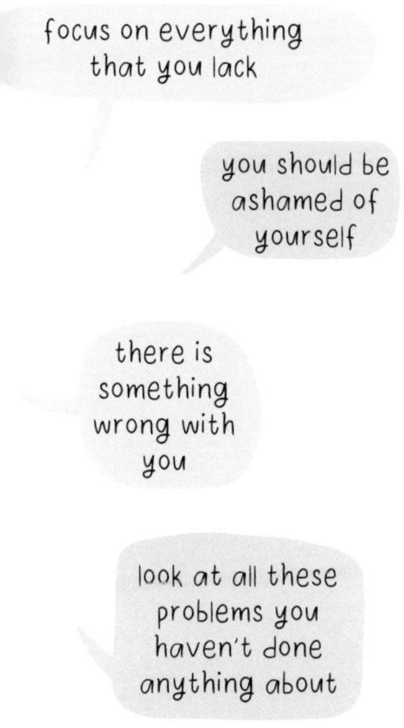
focus on everything that you lack
you should be ashamed of yourself
there is something wrong with you
look at all these problems you haven't done anything about

If I indulged in a decadent treat, the voice would scold me for how 'disgusting' I was, how much self-discipline I lacked.

It took me years to discover that this voice had a name: the inner critic. When I started my recovery journey, I understood that if I wanted to get better, that voice had to go. I needed something louder, something kinder, to stand up against my relentless inner critic.

In 2016, I had been in therapy for a few years, and felt like I was at a standstill; I wasn't making progress at the pace I was used to. My then-therapist invited me to a group therapy treatment with the theme 'self-compassion'. This term was new to me, but I loved going to groups so I signed up, unaware at the time that it would change my life. Without self-compassion in my toolkit, the best instrument to finally silence the inner critic, I don't think I could have worked towards feeling better.

The first group meeting started with an explanation of what self-compassion means.

Compassion is a feeling caused by noticing suffering or

SELF-COMPASSION
COMING TOGETHER

self-kindness

mindfulness

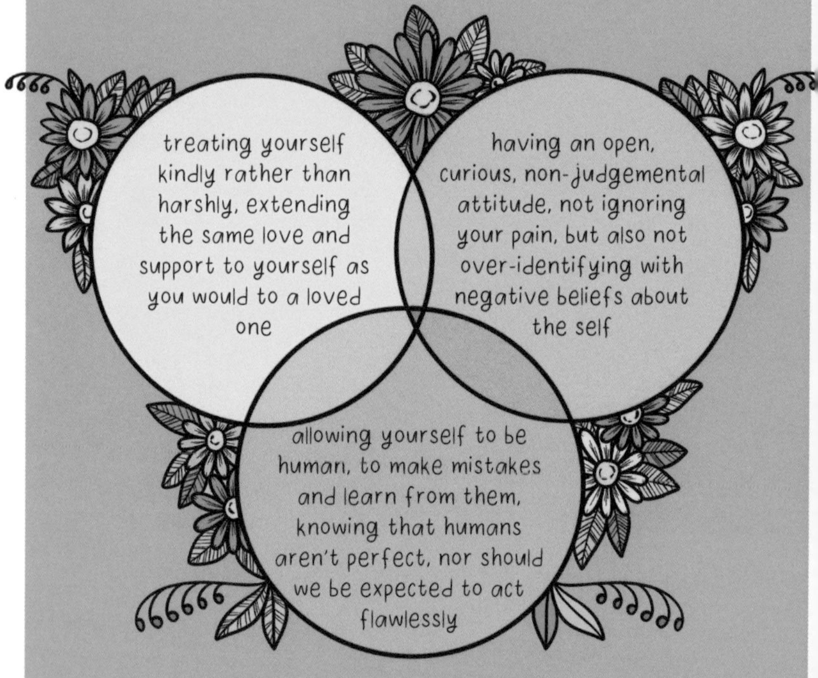

treating yourself kindly rather than harshly, extending the same love and support to yourself as you would to a loved one

having an open, curious, non-judgemental attitude, not ignoring your pain, but also not over-identifying with negative beliefs about the self

allowing yourself to be human, to make mistakes and learn from them, knowing that humans aren't perfect, nor should we be expected to act flawlessly

common humanity

pain in others and reacting to it with warmth. Self-compassion means we respond to our own pain, failures or perceived flaws with the same tenderness and care that we'd give others. The psychologist Dr Kristin Neff has identified three things that allow us to do this: self-kindness (treating ourselves kindly), mindfulness (an open, non-judgmental attitude to our thoughts and feelings) and common humanity (allowing yourself to be an imperfect human, like others).

Sounds easy, but it proved harder than I thought. We did a joint guided meditation and

I remember feeling uncomfortable keeping my eyes closed in a room full of strangers. They let us pick a bracelet from a basket and told us to put it on, and for every negative thought we had, we would switch the bracelet from one wrist to the other. This would raise our awareness of the things we tell ourselves, so that we could start to recognize when we were treating ourselves with compassion and when we weren't. I moved my bracelet so often at first, one of my friends asked me once if I was 'praying or something'.

This group made me realize two important things about myself: one, my first reaction to making mistakes or falling short was always

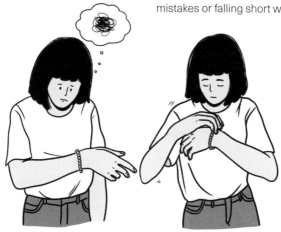

self-criticism and judgment; and two, I would do just about anything to avoid acknowledging my suffering, because then I'd have to deal with it, and I didn't know how to. Instead, a negative thought would turn up and I'd push it away, only for another one to arrive soon after.

This cheap plastic bracelet became a symbol of my suffering, in a way. It helped me compartmentalise my negative thoughts, to notice them as just that – negative – not true, but negative. It made me aware of what situations prompted these thoughts. It invited me to try to replace the negative thought with something a little kinder. Instead of letting the thought destroy me,

my thought process went more like, 'Oh, here's another negative thought. Where did that come from, and how can I transform it?'

I started picturing self-compassion as the antithesis of my inner critic. I imagined self-compassion as a friend, my biggest cheerleader, a light inside myself that could shine outwards if I nurtured it from within. I started questioning everything my inner critic said, and replaced any mean thought with a kinder truth.

It's easy to feel isolated in suffering. The human brain is amazing at making us feel like we are alone in our faults and insecurities, like nobody else can really understand.

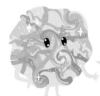

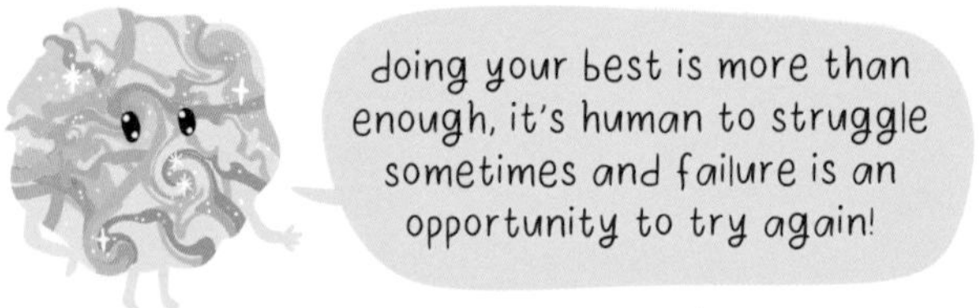

doing your best is more than enough, it's human to struggle sometimes and failure is an opportunity to try again!

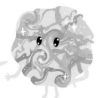

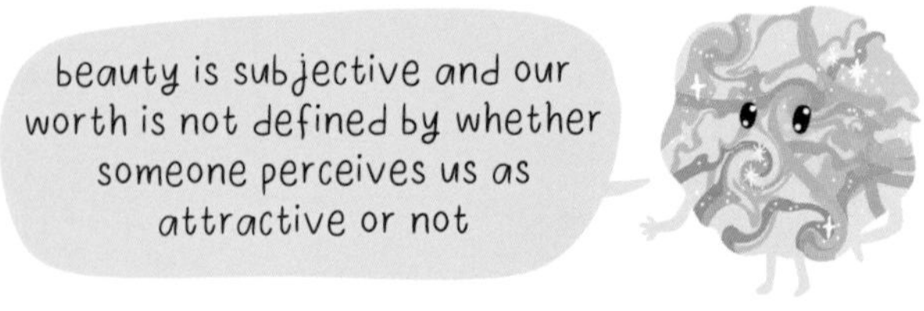

beauty is subjective and our worth is not defined by whether someone perceives us as attractive or not

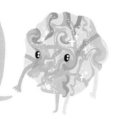

things are hard right now but remember that it doesn't have to be like this forever. focus on making today better with what energy you have. be kind to yourself

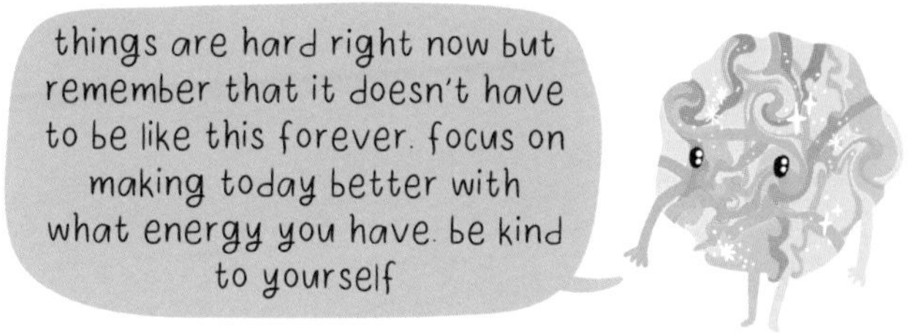

But self-compassion teaches us that our pain and feelings of inadequacy are part of the human experience. This is what differentiates self-compassion from self-pity. In self-compassion, we understand that we're not alone in feeling pain, while self-pity can make us feel like pain and misfortune is somehow targeted and personal. We can notice those thoughts and feelings without letting them consume us. I used to think, 'Why is this happening to me? Why do I have to feel like this?' But now I know it happens to everyone; there is nothing broken about me that needs fixing. My suffering isn't unique, and I find tremendous comfort in that.

Pain connects us if we allow ourselves to be vulnerable. My pain isn't a personal failure in the illusive, endless pursuit of happiness, but a core component of my humanity. That's not to say that we should just accept pain and be miserable, but it's important not to judge ourselves for our suffering, because struggling doesn't mean you are failing, no matter what you have been conditioned to believe.

Sometimes we shame ourselves for feeling bad, assigning personal blame instead of comforting ourselves. When we begin to treat inner pain with tenderness and empathy, we can shift the way we see ourselves through positive change. Self-compassion can serve as a reminder that you deserve the same kindness you'd offer to others, because you are just as worthy as everyone else.

PRACTISING SELF-COMPASSION CAN LOOK LIKE

recognising the voice of your inner critic without judgement, but not getting sucked into negative rumination. trying to replace the negative thoughts with encouragement

trying one of the many guided meditations from self-compassion.org

meeting yourself where you are and being patient. progress takes time and self-compassion is a skill you can build throughout your life

keeping a journal to use for processing but remembering to write lovingly to yourself instead of harshly - don't judge yourself because of your emotions or thoughts giving yourself room to be human – we all make mistakes and we all have things to work on. give yourself permission to feel things without labelling yourself as bad, wrong, lazy, unproductive, etc.

seeing a moment of suffering as just that, a moment that will pass, a part of being human. then ask yourself what you need to hear and tell it to yourself

treating yourself like you would treat a child or a friend if they were hurt or sad. would you criticize or blame, or would you hold comfort and care for them?

giving yourself permission to meet your own needs! everyone needs to recharge their batteries sometimes

finding a soothing touch to engage your parasympathetic nervous system, like placing a hand on your heart or wrapping your arms around yourself in a gentle squeeze

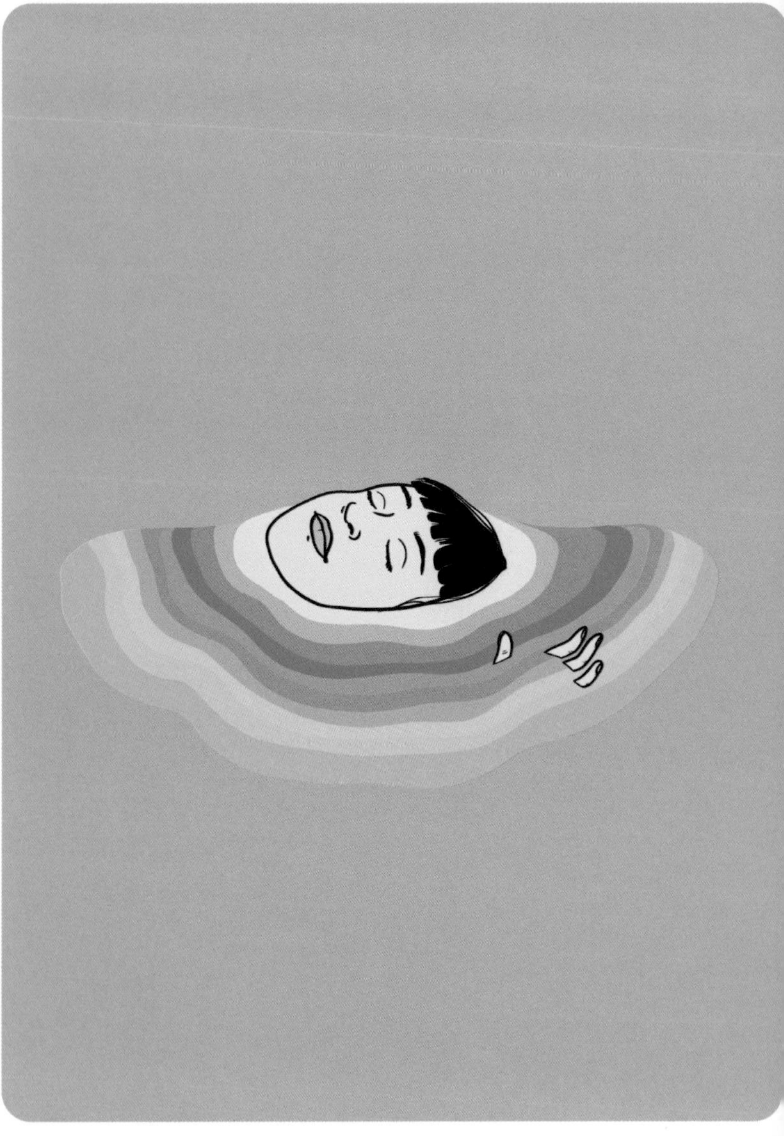

A guide to real self-care

Prioritizing self-care has been a fundamental part of my recovery journey. I'll admit, I used to roll my eyes at it, because I didn't like baths and I didn't fancy having an elaborate skincare routine. The self-care I saw on social media seemed focused on over-indulgence and copious amounts of retail therapy. Then I realized it wasn't about that.

Anything that feeds your soul is self-care. Anything that makes you feel like you did your future self

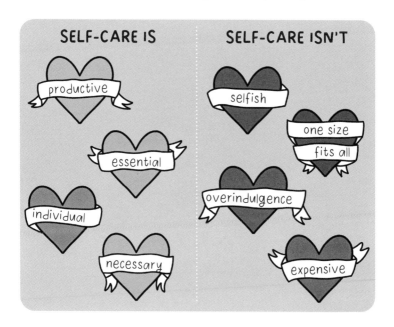

SELF-CARE IS
- productive
- essential
- individual
- necessary

SELF-CARE ISN'T
- selfish
- one size fits all
- overindulgence
- expensive

a favour is self-care, and everything you do to tend to your health and cope with stress is self-care. It doesn't just exist as pampering sessions (although those can be important too!), instead there are many types of self-care activities, as individual as we are. For you, self-care could be spending quality time with yourself doing something creative, meal-prepping for the week ahead, limiting social media consumption, or making plans with someone you love.

Self-care has many benefits. Performing acts of kindness for yourself can help boost your self-esteem. It gives us space away from stress, invites us to devote time to relaxation, can improve our general health and sense of wellbeing, and it reminds us that our health is important.

And since self-care is individual, it's helpful to make a personal plan to fit your needs. Step one could be assessing your current habits and writing a list of the positive and negative coping strategies you have developed over the years. Maybe you are already on top of your practical self-care, but you have been neglecting your emotional self-care. Ask yourself:

- When do I feel the most content?
- What cheers me up when I feel sad?
- What helps me calm down after a stressful day?
- What energizes me when I feel drained?

This should help you understand what helps you and what you may need to do more of, and once you find the gaps you can pick some easy activities to lift your mood in your daily life. Not everyone has the luxury of lots of free time, and fitting in self-care activities can be really hard – so start small (see pages 106–107 for ideas). Adding a quick activity in the morning or evening is a good first step. It's okay for your self-care priorities to change, so check in with yourself regularly and ask yourself what your most urgent need is right now. This will help steer you towards the activity that will help most at a specific time.

SELF-CARE CAN BE ...

social self-care

keeping in touch with friends

calling or texting someone you care about

activities that help us nurture our relationships and maintain our social bonds

getting involved in a social activity in your community

communicating your wants, needs and boundaries

joining an online support group

establishing a support system

spiritual self-care

volunteering in your community

going to your place of worship or your safe place

connecting with nature through mindful walking

activities that nurture our spirit and allow us to connect with something bigger than ourselves

trying yoga or doing some stretching

meditating or praying

dedicating time for self-reflection

CONTINUED ...

SELF-CARE CAN BE ...

mental self-care

activities that stimulate and fascinate our minds and intellect

- listening to an interesting podcast
- visiting a cultural sight in your city
- learning something new
- solving a crossword, puzzle, sudoku, etc.
- reading a book
- playing a board game or a video game

emotional self-care

caring for our emotional needs by identifying, processing and nurturing our feelings

- attending therapy or talking about your feelings with someone
- practising mindfulness when you feel overwhelmed
- trying a guided meditation
- journalling
- creating art
- practising gratitude

practical self-care

completing essential daily tasks that help us prevent stress and make our days easier

- household chores like laundry, dishes, cleaning, etc.
- scheduling and planning
- organising and decluttering
- setting realistic goals for the week ahead
- meal-prepping
- budgeting

physical self-care

activities that promote and nurture the body's general health and hygiene

- practising healthy sleep hygiene
- taking care of your sexual health
- moving your body in ways that feel good to you
- brushing your teeth, washing your hands, bathing or showering
- staying hydrated and nourished
- checking in with your body's needs

BUILDING A SELF-CARE ROUTINE

start small by implementing some easy self-care activities into your daily life, then add in more activities once the original acts start feeling like habits. pick and choose, and ignore the ones that don't feel relevant to your life. replace them with ones that do!

MORNING

do some quick stretching

drink a big glass of water

five minute guided meditation

text someone you love a 'good morning!'

think of three things you're grateful for

make or pick up a filling breakfast

set a daily intention

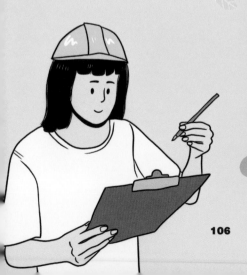

AFTERNOON

tell yourself an affirmation

listen to your favourite song

check in with yourself – press pause and have a moment of reflection

have a snack you feel excited about

take some deep breaths

do a random act of kindness

declutter for ten minutes

EVENING

prepare for tomorrow

put your phone away for a bit

look up some positive news

change into your coziest clothes

catch up with someone you care about

write a quick brain dump

take a moment to unwind before you go to bed

Building boundaries

Boundaries are the lines we draw between us and others. Together, they build up our agency, our personal limits. We need personal boundaries to have respectful and healthy relationships with other people – and ourselves too – and this is why they are crucial to better mental health.

I wasn't very good at boundaries until recently. As a kid and teen I didn't have lots of friends, so I felt that I needed to always be agreeable and available, otherwise I might lose them. So I typically went along with others, said yes to things I didn't really care for and put myself last. It wasn't until I realized that my lack of boundaries was making me resentful of people in my life – people that hadn't really done anything wrong, they just couldn't read my mind.

Meeting my first boyfriend taught me a lot about boundaries. He noticed pretty early on that I didn't have a lot of them and tended towards being people-pleasing. He reminded me of my right to choose through small acts, like asking when I had time to see him, asking my likes and dislikes, by having his own boundaries and reminding me of them by reacting to boundaries with respect and understanding. Being close to someone who gave me agency and space in the relationship helped me set boundaries with other people too. It started with small things at first, like saying, 'I have to hang up the phone now, talk to you later', or, 'I really don't like that restaurant – would you mind if we went somewhere else?'. Other people's reactions to my boundaries became an early test of compatibility for me. If someone couldn't respect my boundaries, I distanced myself from them, and soon I found myself surrounded with strong bonds and by people who I felt secure to be myself around.

CREATING AND ASSERTING BOUNDAIRES

think about what your basic human rights are. it can be things like ...

- the right to decide what to do with your time
- the right to be treated with respect
- the right to say no without feeling bad

ask yourself what your values are, what makes you uncomfortable, what makes you feel disrespected?

think about what you want to accomplish with your boundaries and how best to react if someone rejects them

listen to your gut instinct, really tune into how you feel

communicate with others, be direct and assertive

set appropriate consequences to any boundary violations and let people know those consequences

start small and build your boundaries as your relationships progress

make sure your boundaries aren't too rigid as a subconscious effort to keep others at a distance

remember that it's okay for boundaries to change over time and that you can have different boundaries with different people

be consistent with your boundaries and practice saying no and speaking your mind often

MY BOUNDARIES

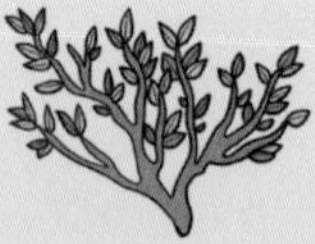

i will communicate
any discomfort
i feel

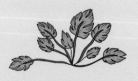

i will not allow others
to guilt-trip me, and
i won't be pressured
into things i'm
uncomfortable with

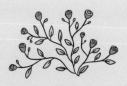

i will not sacrifice
my emotional
needs

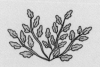

i will stand up for
myself and voice
my opinions with
confidence

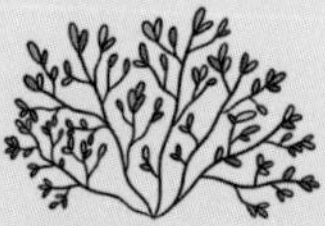

i will not hold myself
responsible for
things beyond
my control

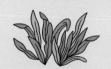

i will communicate
openly and, when
i need to,
assertively

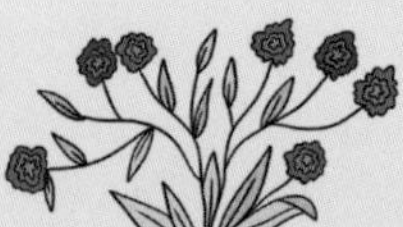

i will not let my
happiness depend
on other people's
opinions

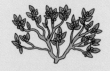

i will prioritize my
mental health and
physical wellbeing

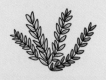

i will step away from
people who make
me feel small and
inadequate

It can be hard to know how to establish boundaries. Maybe you feel unsure about expressing your needs and limits. Perhaps you grew up feeling like your autonomy wasn't respected, or that your voice wasn't listened to. Learning your boundaries means asking yourself what you need to feel safe and heard, and enforcing those boundaries. This can take a lot of bravery at first, but everytime you uphold a boundary, it will help you build your confidence and sense of self.

BOUNDARIES CAN SOUND LIKE

i don't feel comfortable sharing about that so let's drop it now

i am not interested so please don't ask me again

i have to leave early tonight, just so you know

i don't accept people yelling at me so if you don't stop i will leave this conversation

i don't like being touched in that way so don't do that again

i want to help but i don't have much time right now and i dont want to overextend. is there another time we could do this?

don't go into my room without knocking first

you can't borrow my car tomorrow, i need it for an appointment

i need some space for myself tonight, let's hang out soon though

please don't make jokes like that around me, it makes me uncomfortable

Managing negative thoughts

there's no point in trying

i'm gonna fail like i always do

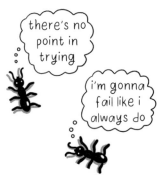

When I was 15, I developed social anxiety disorder. I was never a shy kid, but starting at a brand new school for the first time stripped all sense of safety away – making me increasingly aware of how difficult it can be to make a good first impression. I was already dealing with my out-of-control generalized anxiety disorder, so this really was the cherry on top. The social anxiety disorder was missed when I first went to therapy, because my generalized anxiety masked it. If something scared me, I avoided it. The more I avoided things, the more frightening it all seemed, and that was the circle I became stuck in.

During the worst of it, I must have gone a whole year without thinking a single positive thing about myself. The way I made sense of the world was through a lens of negativity, because it all felt hopeless. My social anxiety fed off these negative thoughts and fears, and my brain rewarded me for listening to negativity; when I avoided what scared me, the social anxiety part of my brain felt safe and satiated.

i can't do anything right

bad things always happen to me

i'm not worthy

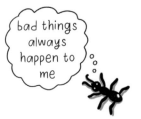

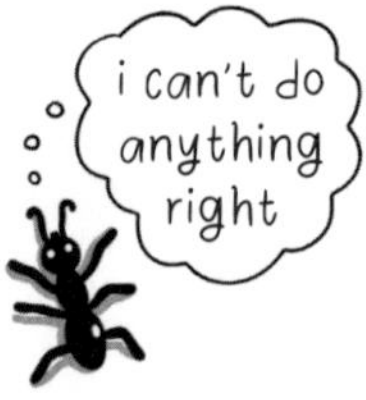

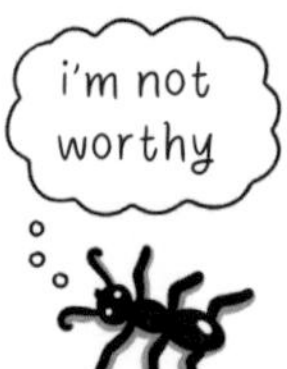

this is all my fault

i'm never gonna be happy again

I like to imagine our brains as big forests with millions of little paths. Each path symbolizes a thought, and these paths – as they run in parallel, stretch away from each other, and sometimes converge – form patterns just as our thoughts connect and build on each other. When we think of something new, we form a new little path where there wasn't one before. The more we think about a specific thought, the more established and walkable the path becomes, and therefore we subconsciously choose to walk on that path again and again. The paths of thoughts we push aside become overgrown and unwalkable, until it's like they never existed.

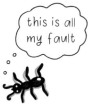

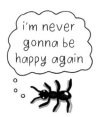

If we think of a negative thought again and again, it becomes a main road and seems all the more truthful. As we learned in Chapter 2, our thoughts form habits and beliefs, and go onto inform the way we see ourselves and the world, for better or worse.

When I was in the midst of social anxiety disorder, I let my negative thoughts bulldoze over any positive thoughts that were there before. My forest had gone from a vast, beautiful reserve to a loud, littered, cemented construction site of negativity – and it was up to me to restore it to what it was before.

In the self-compassion course I did, I learnt about automatic negative thoughts (shortened to ANTs), and the link between social anxiety and negative thinking patterns.

When confronted with ANTs, our best bet is to challenge them. The goal is to gently remind ourselves that our negative

nobody Cares about me

i'm just a bad person after all

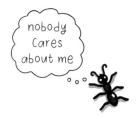

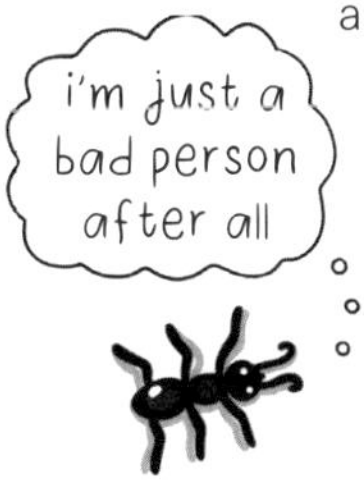

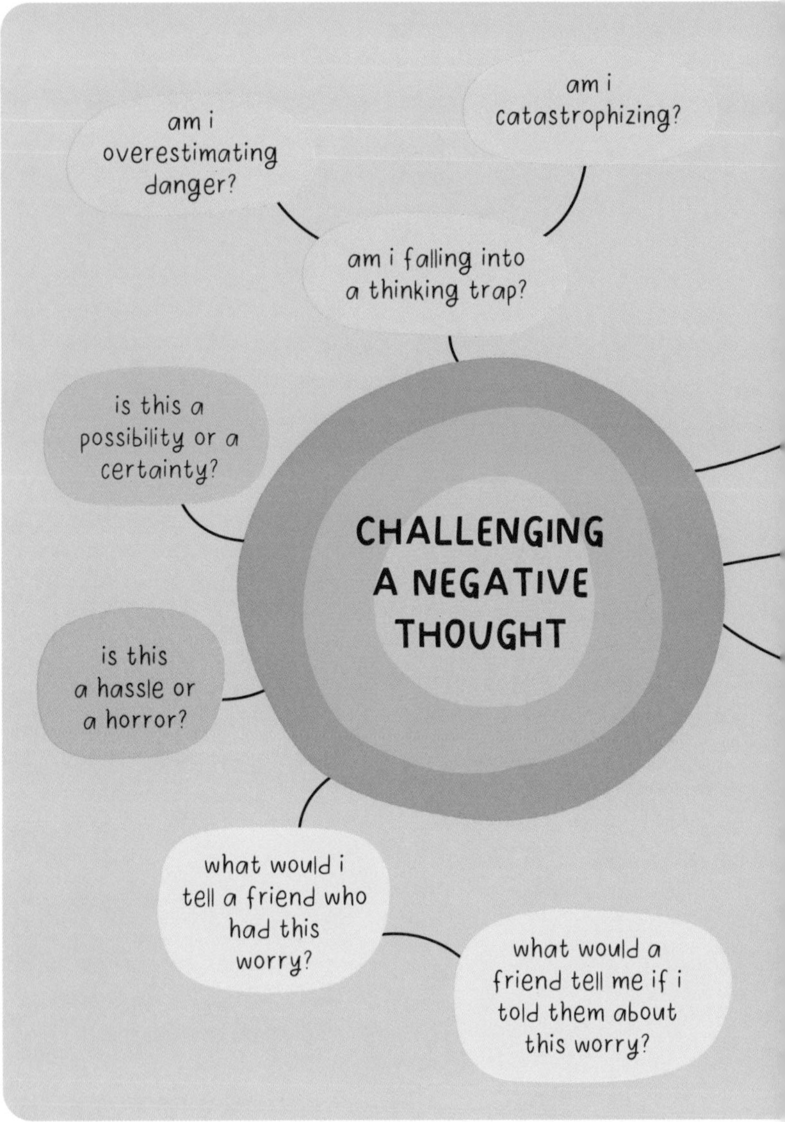
CHALLENGING A NEGATIVE THOUGHT
am i falling into a thinking trap?
am i overestimating danger?
am i catastrophizing?
is this a possibility or a certainty?
is this a hassle or a horror?
what would i tell a friend who had this worry?
what would a friend tell me if i told them about this worry?

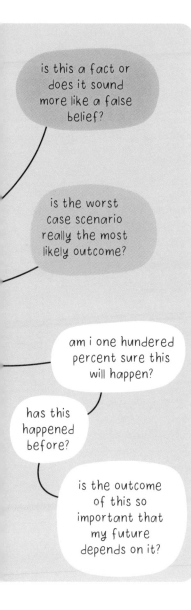

is this a fact or does it sound more like a false belief?

is the worst case scenario really the most likely outcome?

am i one hundered percent sure this will happen?

has this happened before?

is the outcome of this so important that my future depends on it?

thoughts are often not an accurate reflection of our reality, and are more telling of the way we see ourselves.

So what do we do once we've challenged our negative thoughts? We replace the ANTs with PETs (positive empowering thoughts). I welcome you to try this simple exercise, writing down your own negative thoughts, and finding positive ones to take their place.

- Get a pen and paper; find a quiet place to reflect. Draw two columns.
- Take a moment to calm your mind; breathe in and out slowly.
- Ask yourself, what negative things am I telling myself? Write them down in the first column, not worrying about spelling or grammar.
- Next, consider each thought in turn and ask yourself, honestly, how could I challenge this and turn it into a positive thought? Write the positives down in the next column.

The next time you find yourself in a negative thought spiral, you can look back at your positive and empowering thoughts instead.

Coping, grounding and soothing

We all need ways to cope with difficult circumstances. I like to think of 'coping' as being able to adjust and minimize stress, and tolerate negative or painful emotions. It can be conscious or unconscious, and not all coping strategies are created equal.

Before I learnt about healthy coping mechanisms, I coped in unhealthy ways. When I was anxious, I coped by avoiding whatever was making me worried. When I felt traumatized by really difficult experiences, I coped by restricting my food as a way to regain control of my body. When I was struck with really painful emotions, I coped by smoking cigarettes or drinking alcohol.

It took me a long time to realize that behaviours that made me feel better in the moment, but which didn't make a positive change in the long run, weren't effective coping strategies. Sometimes we carry so much with us, it's hard to know what we need to heal from, and sometimes, as we're working actively on our healing, more and more inner wounds are uncovered. In the moments when emotional pain catches us off guard, having healthy coping skills comes in handy.

There are hundreds of ways to cope, but they can all be divided into two categories: problem-based coping and emotion-based coping. Some negative feelings can be resolved or relieved by problem-based coping, like saying 'no' to a social obligation that you don't want to do in the first place, instead of saying 'yes' to appease others at the cost of your time and energy.

Emotion-based coping is helpful for times where the anxiety and stress come from

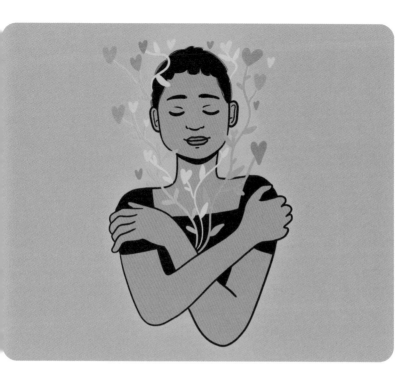

circumstances beyond our control, like when we're dealing with loss or illness, for example. This method of coping could include doing a mediation exercise, or journaling to take some time to reflect and regulate your feelings.

These methods can also be used together, like if you have a job interview that you're really anxious about, problem-based coping could be researching the company beforehand and prepping answers to feel more prepared, and emotion-based coping could be thinking of affirmations to tell yourself before the interview to make yourself feel more confident.

What I love about coping skills is that they can be tailored to fit your individual needs, and I truly believe that there's a coping skill for every problem I might face. So the next time you feel sad, stressed

SOME WAYS TO COPE

creative pursuits, like writing, drawing or photography

listen to music

tend to your plants or garden

singing, dancing, playing an instrument

visualize a calm, happy and safe place

reward or pamper yourself

engage your body in exercise

cry it out

call someone you trust

eat something you have been craving

identify three things you like about yourself

journal about it

communicate your needs

watch something that makes you laugh

stretch

bake or cook something

read a book or watch a movie or a TV series

try a yoga breathing exercise

pet an animal

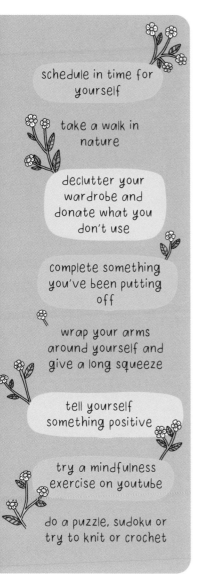

schedule in time for yourself

take a walk in nature

declutter your wardrobe and donate what you don't use

complete something you've been putting off

wrap your arms around yourself and give a long squeeze

tell yourself something positive

try a mindfulness exercise on youtube

do a puzzle, sudoku or try to knit or crochet

or angry, set aside a moment to try a new coping technique.

Some coping strategies involve grounding techniques. Grounding techniques are ways to connect to your body when you're trapped in your head. They bring you back to the present moment when you're struck by strong emotions or traumatic memories.

At the height of my PTSD and panic disorder I would dissociate often: my hands and feet would go completely numb and sometimes I felt like an uninvited stranger in my own body. Dissociating was my brain's way of protecting me from pain, but as it stopped access to pain, it also stopped access to healing. Learning how to 'come back down to earth' was essential for unlocking my ability to work through those emotions.

Grounding is a way to bring us back into the present. I like to see it as bringing the consciousness from inside your mind to meet with an awareness of your body.

For some people, grounding can be spiritual in nature, but grounding has a therapeutic and biological basis. When we are

GROUNDING TECHNIQUES

think in categories. choose topics like 'animals' or 'names of colours' and list as many as you can

name five things you can see, four things you can feel, three things you can hear, two things you can smell and one thing you can taste

put an ice cube in your mouth and let it melt on your tongue

count to a hundred

clench your hands into fists, hold for a few seconds, then release the tension. repeat ten times

put your hands under running water and alternate from warm and cold and feel the different sensations

pick a colour and name all the things around you that are that colour

think of an object and try to 'draw' it in the air with your finger

take ten slow, deep breaths in through your nose and out through your mouth

recite something you know by heart like a song or a poem

eat something slowly and try to savour every bite

stressed, our sympathetic nervous system activates our flight/fight/freeze response to get us ready for facing or avoiding danger. It produces stress hormones like cortisol, which makes us feel anxious and afraid, and gets our heart beating as we produce adrenaline. Grounding helps us activate our parasympathetic nervous system, the 'rest and digest' system, which makes us calm and relaxed again. Here's a simple way to test this out yourself: the next time you are stressed, exhale for twice as long as you inhale for each breath you take – this tells our body that we are safe and ready to calm down.

Soothing is a similar copying strategy to grounding, in that it makes us feel better in moments of overwhelm. Crying is a perfect example of soothing: it may be one of the body's best mechanisms for self-soothing, a natural ability we form as soon as we are born. As babies, we get soothed in various ways. Now, as an adult, I use similar ways to soothe myself. Instead of being swaddled in a baby blanket, I wrap myself in covers and blankets. I listen to calming music and guided meditations when I'm trying to go to sleep but have an anxious mind. I rock back and forth with my eyes shut, feet planted on the ground, focusing on my breathing. When I'm in need of soothing, I keep my inner-child in mind: what does she need to feel safe?

If you want to add these coping techniques to your self-care toolkit, take a moment to think about ways you could self-soothe, and what types of grounding techniques you'd like to try. Maybe think back to a moment when you felt safe or comforted, and identify what brought you peace in that moment. Write down some of the things that cause you stress, then, next to them, write down activities, exercises or methods for coping that you can have on hand and use when you need to. Set aside a moment at the end of your day to practice a self-soothing habit. Taking some time in the evening to ground yourself can make it easier to process the day's events and feel more peaceful as you get ready to sleep.

Breathing
and mindfulness

I must confess, the first time that someone suggested I should try breathing exercises for my anxiety, I felt a bit patronized, and most likely responded with something snarky like, 'I already know how to breathe, otherwise I'd be dead right?' I wasn't convinced something as simple as breathing could do anything in terms of feeling better.

It wasn't until years later, when I had gone from my early teens to late teens, and had a really intense panic attack, that I finally caved and tried a breathing exercise called 'box breathing'. To my surprise, my panic attack started to subdue faster than ever before. This is because when we do breathwork exercises, we activate the body's parasympathetic nervous system (more about this on page 119–121). From that moment, I started researching the science behind mindful

breathing, and now it's one of my most dependable coping skills. Breathwork has been the simplest, most easily accessible, and fastest-working activity to help calm me down that I've ever used. You can do it anytime, anywhere and throughout the day.

Mindfulness is another thing that also changed my life; I started actively practising mindfulness after learning about it in the self-compassion course I did. Mindfulness is the practice of bringing yourself back into the present moment without being overwhelmed or reactive, allowing a moment-by-moment awareness of our physical sensations, thoughts, and feelings, without judgment. When I feel emotionally drained, mindfulness is like rechanging my internal battery. The benefits of mindfulness are vast: improvement of general health, enhanced ability to deal with negative emotions, and decreased stress, to name a few. I think every person could benefit from incorporating mindfulness into their lives. An easy way to incorporate mindfulness is to fall asleep to a guided meditation.

I listen to a video on YouTube and it helps quiet my busy mind, and it makes me feel safe as I enter sleep. There are many ways of practicing both breathwork and mindfulness, and one of my favourite exercises for both is the box breath.

BOX BREATH

Sit quietly, and become aware of the natural rhythm of your breath, without changing it at all.

Then, consciously breathe in slowly, to the count of four:
(in) 1, 2, 3, 4.
Do this without changing how you naturally breathe out.

After a few breaths like this, breathe in to the count of four, and breathe out to the count of four:
(in) 1, 2, 3, 4 (out) 1, 2, 3, 4.

After a few breaths of in on the count of four, and out on the count of four, pause at the top for a count of four:
(in) 1, 2, 3, 4 (pause) 1, 2, 3, 4 (out) 1, 2, 3, 4.

After a few breaths like this, pause for a count of four after you have breathed out:
(in) 1, 2, 3, 4 (pause) 1, 2, 3, 4
(out) 1, 2, 3, 4 (pause) 1, 2, 3, 4
(in) 1, 2, 3, 4 *and so on.*
This is the box breath.

Do this for a few more box breaths, then gradually begin to breathe normally. Gently waken your body by wiggling your toes and fingers, before being ready to return to your day.

Processing in words

The power of putting words to your feelings is immense. Processing what's wrong typically begins after we put it into words, and after that we can start to work through it.

There are many mental health benefits of journaling: it helps create awareness, can bring us out of rumination, helps us practice opening up and being vulnerable

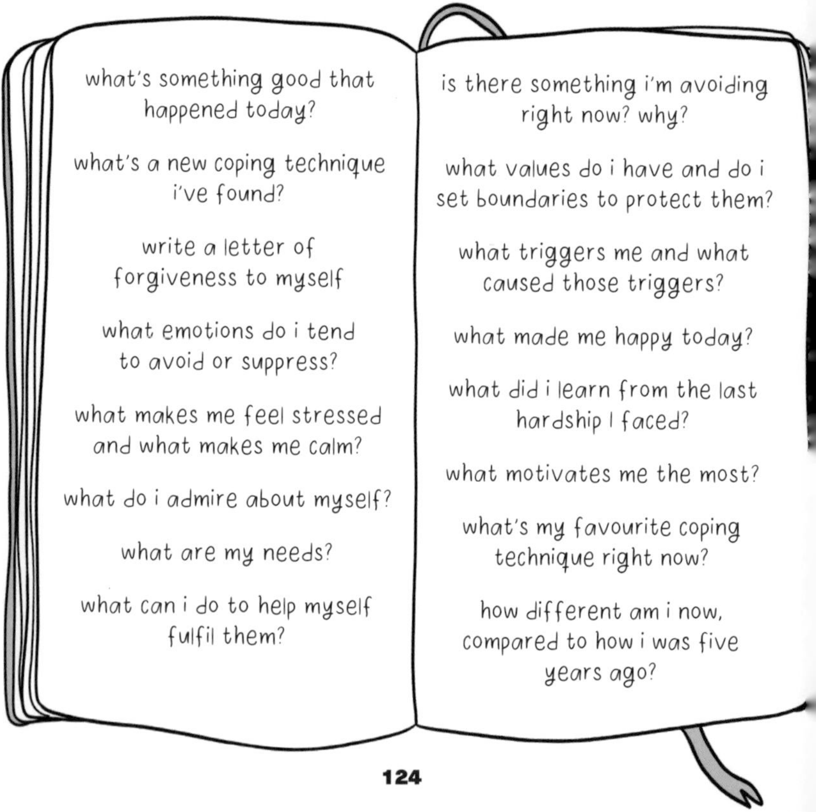
what's something good that happened today?
what's a new coping technique i've found?
write a letter of forgiveness to myself
what emotions do i tend to avoid or suppress?
what makes me feel stressed and what makes me calm?
what do i admire about myself?
what are my needs?
what can i do to help myself fulfil them?
is there something i'm avoiding right now? why?
what values do i have and do i set boundaries to protect them?
what triggers me and what caused those triggers?
what made me happy today?
what did i learn from the last hardship I faced?
what motivates me the most?
what's my favourite coping technique right now?
how different am i now, compared to how i was five years ago?

with our feelings, and reduces stress. If you search for 'mental health journal prompts' there's an abundance of suggestions.

Talking about feelings allows you to acknowledge them, opens the door for others to support you, and can help you work through them. Sometimes it's hard to even know what we really feel until we start talking about it, and it all becomes clearer. Healthy emotional venting is a great tool for processing feelings.

It can be hard to open up if we didn't grow up being taught how to discuss emotions, so it can be a learning curve at first, which is why journaling can be a first step to opening up, before talking to someone like a friend, family member or teacher at school.

One of the most important foundations of healing, and of maintaining good mental health in general, is other people. Having a support system and not feeling like you're on your own is a lifeline for many. Take a moment to think about the people in your life: do you feel like you can talk to them, or that you are there for each other when times get hard?

What do you do if you feel like you don't have anyone like that? Maybe you struggle to make friends, or grew up in a family where you weren't allowed to be vulnerable, or perhaps you are finding yourself in a new place without anyone to lean on. If this is your current reality, there are places and ways to connect with others and start to build a support system for yourself.

It can be scary to make friends, especially if you have struggled with bullying or feelings of isolation in the past. Many people find it hard to put themselves out there, so you're not alone in feeling daunted about forming new connections. But you'd be surprised how many people would love to have a friend like you, and how many people crave that same need for support. Finding groups and activities that interest you is a big help for making natural connections with like-minded people. Looking locally for free events or cheap classes/courses is a good first step. If you have people in your life with large friend groups, try to link up with them. Making friends is a process, but remember that the worst thing that could happen is that you find you might not be compatible as friends, and that's okay, because you can try again. It gets easier with time: vulnerability is something you have to practice to get more comfortable with.

Therapy is another place to open up about feelings in a safe and controlled way.

FINDING COMMUNITY AND CONNECTION

research local events

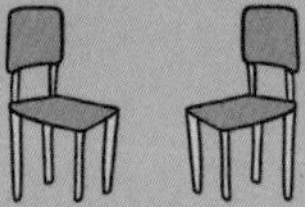

seek out a support group

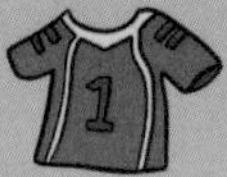
1

join a sports team

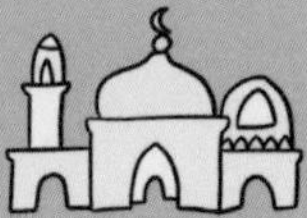

visit a place of worship

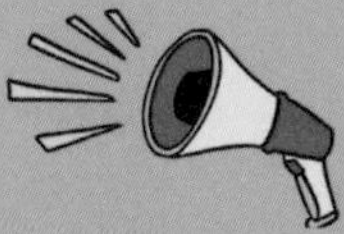

look for advocacy or volunteer work

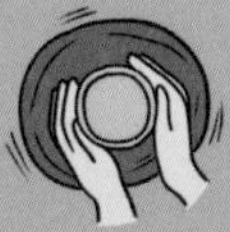

try out a beginner class like pottery, or a language course

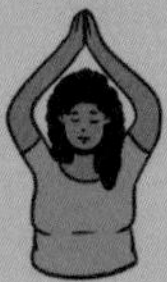

try a yoga or dance class

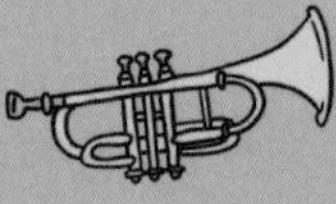

join or start a band or creative endevour

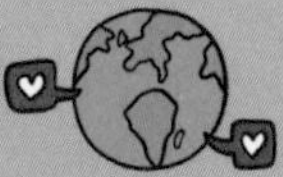

find online communities with shared interests

TIPS ON MAKING FRIENDS

make yourself available by going to places and events where other people are

try to form deeper connections with casual acquaintances

practice talking to people, compliment others and strike up casual conversations whenever you can

get to know the friends of people you already know

be curious and attentive when talking to people. smiling and showing interest goes a long way!

be yourself! making real friends depends on you daring to be vulnerable and authentically you

think about what qualities are important to you in a friend, then practice exemplifying those qualities

be consistent and put effort into staying in touch, even in small ways like a quick text

work on your confidence: it's all about practice. it's scary to initiate a 'friend date', but everyone needs a friend, and other people feel just as nervous as you do!

Unfortunately, in most places, therapy is a privilege not afforded to all. However, there are different strategies for finding therapy for free or cheap, depending on where you live. See the resources listed on page 190 to learn more about what options might be available to you in terms of therapy, as well as numbers to call if you need to talk to someone.

if you have the option based on your location, research the therapists that best suit your needs. do you need a trauma-informed therapist? An LGBTQIA-informed therapist? A black or POC therapist?

don't be afraid to ask your therapist questions if anything is unclear, or to let them know if something isn't working for you

be honest! your therapist has most likely seen it all. there's nothing too shameful or taboo to talk about in therapy

you might not be sure about your therapist at first, but give it a chance. remember that it's okay to switch therapists if you dont feel like it's a good fit for your needs

it's okay to cry in sessions

make a list of topics to go over, or keep a journal with therapy thoughts that you can bring to your sessions if you forget what to say when you're there

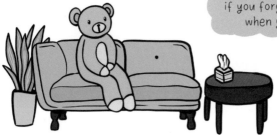

remember that your therapist is there to help you and has your best interest at heart

therapy can bring up a lot of upsetting emotions, so be kind to yourself in between sessions and practice self-care

be prepared to step out of your comfort zone, but don't hesitate to let your therapist know your fears and worries. you are allowed to set the pace, always

go into therapy with an open mind. some exercises might seem silly or pointless at first, but try to be open to trying things genuinely

be patient and realistic with your expectations. Therapy is hard work, and it might take a while before you start to see the fruition of positive change

reflect on your session after it's done. what did you take away from it? how can you apply what you've learnt to your daily life?

think about what you wish to get out of therapy and work with your therapist to set goals

nothing is too 'small' to bring up. it's okay to discuss everyday problems and stressors

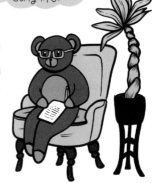

be present during the sessions. don't worry about the time or the things you're saying

What's in your toolkit?

Now that you've looked through my toolkit, I'm inviting you to start building your own. Mental-health work can often be tiring and hard, but a lot of it can be fun and fulfilling, as finding joy is a big part of the journey.

My biggest tip for building your own toolkit is to give everything a try, because sometimes we can be surprised at what works for us. Below is a list where you can check off what you'd like to try implementing in your toolkit!

- ☐ Show compassion to yourself
- ☐ Learn how to really care for yourself
- ☐ Set your boundaries
- ☐ Change your negative thoughts into positive ones
- ☐ Challenge your inner critic
- ☐ Build up healthy coping strategies
- ☐ Learn to ground yourself in the moment
- ☐ Talk it out, write it out, cry it out
- ☐ Soothe yourself

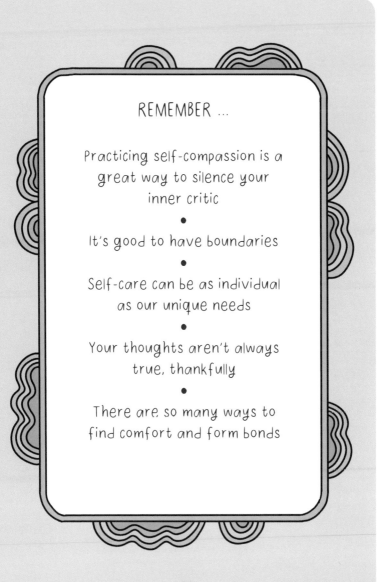

REMEMBER ...

Practicing self-compassion is a great way to silence your inner critic

•

It's good to have boundaries

•

Self-care can be as individual as our unique needs

•

Your thoughts aren't always true, thankfully

•

There are so many ways to find comfort and form bonds

Chapter 4

THE
ROAD
TO
RECOVERY

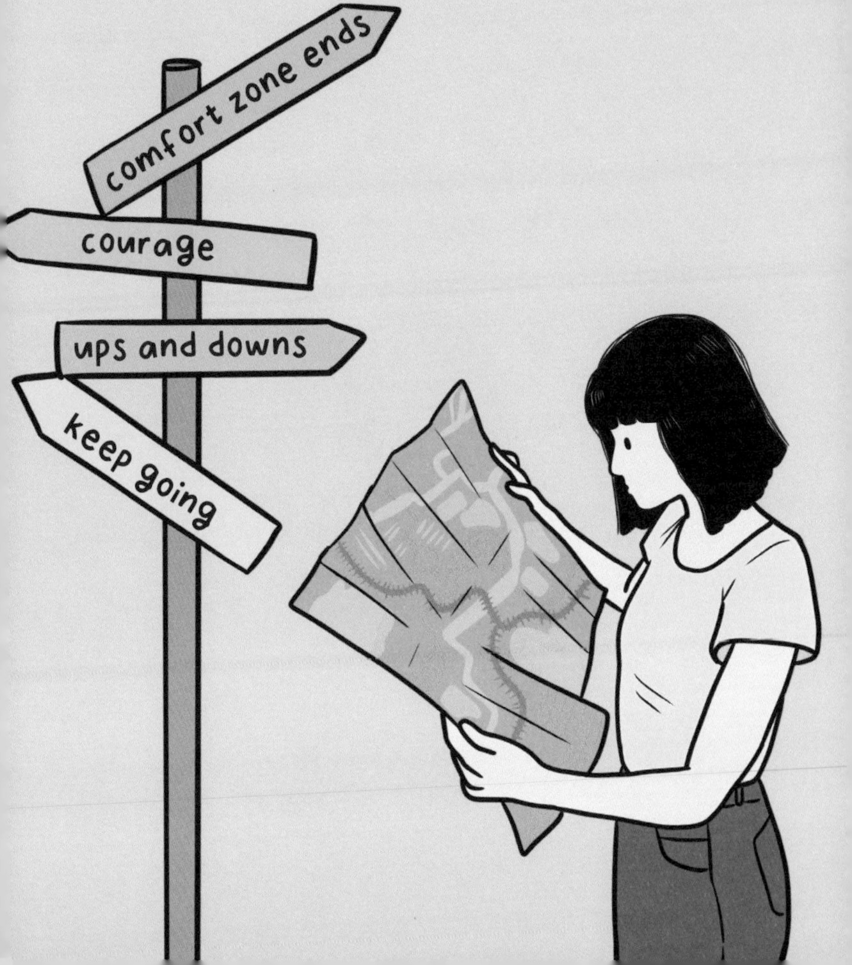
comfort zone ends
courage
ups and downs
keep going

Stress and healing

The road to recovery is rarely smooth – life inevitably throws us curveballs and we have to deal with challenges. Stress is unfortunately a part of life; it's a natural reaction to tough situations. But long-term stress can do a number on our health, as well as set you back when you're trying hard to feel better.

As someone who struggles to regulate my emotions, nothing makes me curl up into a ball on the floor like a stressful day. Stress management has always been a focal point in my therapy treatment, because in the past daily stress impaired my ability to do anything. It triggered panic attacks and depressive episodes, it wreaked

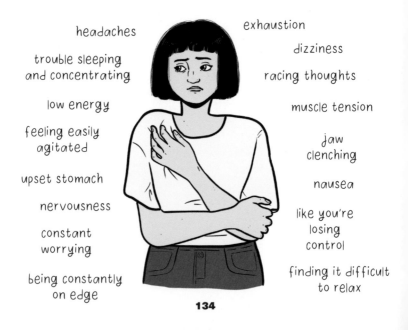

headaches

trouble sleeping
and concentrating

low energy

feeling easily
agitated

upset stomach

nervousness

constant
worrying

being constantly
on edge

exhaustion

dizziness

racing thoughts

muscle tension

jaw
clenching

nausea

like you're
losing
control

finding it difficult
to relax

havoc on my digestive system, I was constantly nauseated and my jaw permanently clenched.

To achieve better mental health, I started looking into ways to prevent stress, arriving at the conclusion that it was time to cut out as many stress triggers I could. If I got an assignment at school that seemed too overwhelming, I marched to my teacher immediately to tell them that I felt stressed and to ask them if they could help me understand what I needed to do. If a day had been stressful, the dishes or the pile of laundry on the floor could wait until tomorrow. If my mornings felt too short, I got up half an hour earlier so I could take my time to wake up without rushing through the first part of my the day.

Look at your routines and daily schedule; take a moment to think about what's causing you stress. Try implementing some of the problem-based or emotion-based coping methods we learned about in the previous chapter (on page 116–117), to either cut out/reduce stressors, or to help yourself build stress tolerance and regulate your feelings.

Sometimes we can't cut the stress out completely, but we can try to build in activities that help to manage how it affects us. One late afternoon, after a particularly rough day in high school, my therapist taught me how to perform body scans. It's akind of meditation that is perfectly suited for beginners. She had me sit comfortably in my chair, eyes closed, and pay attention to each part of my body, piece by piece. I looked out for discomfort, pain or tension, and visualized letting go of it as I moved on. Try it for yourself:

- Get comfortable, sitting or lying down, and close your eyes.
- Listen to your breathing.
- How do your feet feel? Your legs? Your tummy?
- Work your way up your body to the crown of your head, noticing sensations, acknowledging them, letting the thought go.
- And, finally, check in with your emotions. How are you feeling right now?
- Check in with your breathing again – and then let the feelings go.

STRESS PREVENTION

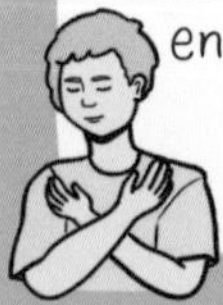

take care of your body with enough sleep, nutrients, water and physical movement

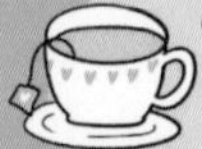

make time for a moment of calm at the end of your evenings

sort the stress in your life into categories:

1. things that can be solved with practical solutions,
2. things that can be solved by asking for help
3. and things you can't control

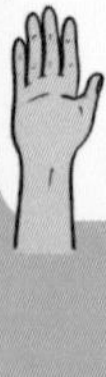

practice saying no to additional responsibilities if you're already busy with your own tasks

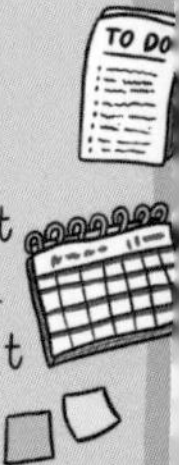
TO DO

organize your tasks in writing. break down big tasks into smaller steps, and lay them out in order of importance. put reminders up on post its, etc. find the task planning system that works for you

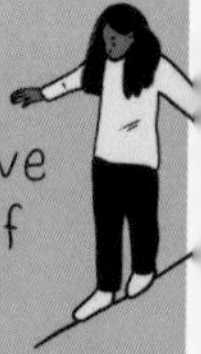

ask yourself: do i have a healthy balance of responsibilities and leisure activities? does my schedule allow for rest? what can i remove or move around to make sure i have time for things to look forward to?

talk about your stress with others and reach out for help if things feel unmanageable

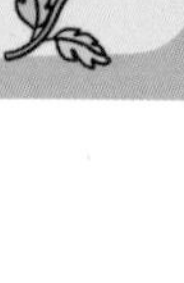

I made it a habit to do body scans whenever I felt stressed. If I noticed pain in my neck, I imagined the pain as a bodily manifestation of my stress and tended to it with tiger balm or a hot compress. Just the act of tending to my own stress in a physical way made me feel more in control of the stress itself.

There's an infinite number of ways to combat stress, and it can be individualized for anyone. It's helpful to plan for potential stress before it happens, to avoid feeling struck by it when it comes. Keeping a list of ways to calm yourself can make you feel more prepared and in control of your emotions.

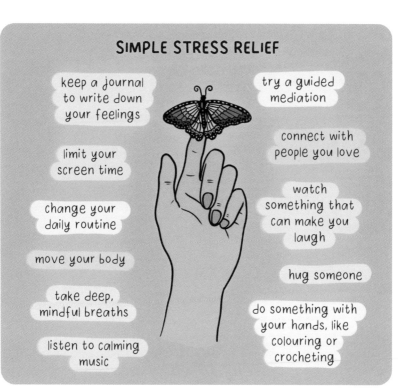

SIMPLE STRESS RELIEF

- keep a journal to write down your feelings
- limit your screen time
- change your daily routine
- move your body
- take deep, mindful breaths
- listen to calming music
- try a guided mediation
- connect with people you love
- watch something that can make you laugh
- hug someone
- do something with your hands, like colouring or crocheting

Coping with productivity frenzy

am i doing enough?

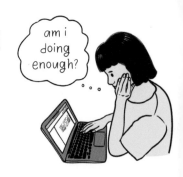

Have you ever been made to feel lazy? Do you struggle to relax and unwind, because you could always do more? Does it feel impossible for you to feel good about a day where you feel you didn't get 'enough done'? Do you feel guilty taking time for yourself because you could spend it working or being productive?

am i doing enough?

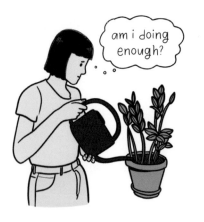

The pressure to overwork is woven into the fabric of our society. Call it what you want – 'the grindset', 'hustle culture' – over-committing and over-extending ourselves has become the norm, and these expectations aren't sound. We are encouraged to place productivity over balance, to the detriment of our health. Scientific studies have shown again and again how we overestimate how long the average person can focus on a task. Our window for attentive productivity is actually only a couple of consecutive hours. So we have brains that work best in short bouts of productivity, but our school/work schedules expect us to stay on task for hours and hours in a row, often for five days a week with inadequate breaks. And at home there are numerous other tasks to be completed.

All of this can compound to make us feel that we are never doing enough, and some of us are prone to reacting to that with 'productivity frenzy' – putting our mental health needs aside, in order to have as much time to do as much as we possibly can. But by ignoring our minds and bodies when they are telling us to slow down, we increase the risk of burnout and poor mental health.

I don't believe in laziness – I believe in situational constraints that make us feel lazy.

Can you not get out of bed

am i doing enough?

am i doing enough?

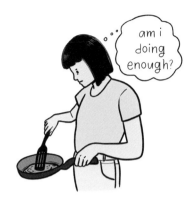

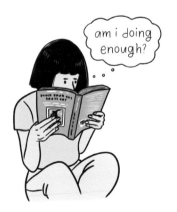

because you're lazy, or do you feel exhausted and drained?

Can you not get your essay done because you're lazy, or because you have five other essays stressing you out?

We have to work to live, we are not fully in control of our time or circumstances, and that can be a tough pill to swallow. And while it's important to try our best to pick a path that is supportive to our mental health, that luxury isn't always available to us, at least not without lots of trial and error. But we do have control of how we measure value in ourselves and others. It's time to let go of the concept that we are only valuable as 'productive members of society', and start to place our self-worth in a way that aligns with our actual priorities. We are just as deserving of our right to exist when we're sitting in bed as we are when we are busy with work; we deserve to feel good about ourselves when we're resting and recharging. We should not feel guilty because we 'could always do more'. Laziness and feelings of demotivation are usually warning signs that we need rest and reprioritize.

I had to take a step back and look at my life, not from the lens of what I'm supposed to want, but what actually matters to me. I saw friends going off to uni and it seemed like the obvious thing to do, but higher education isn't a priority to me. The idea of success is tempting, but I was never an overachiever. I would be content making just enough money to get by if that meant not working as hard, which feels like an ugly thing to admit in a world where it's seen as normal to ask six-year-olds what their future career aspirations are.

I tried keeping as busy as possible when I left school at 19, because I assumed feeling productive would provide a sense of self-satisfaction and make my time feel well-spent. And as I became self-employed I felt the need to monetize everything I did, so I stopped drawing for fun because it 'was a waste of time'. But doing so didn't make me feel better about myself, it made me feel worse. I needed creative play, because it improves my mental health. Balancing my work life and free time helped me feel like I had more control of my life, and taking care of my mental health made work more enjoyable.

Being busy shouldn't define my worth, and I want a life as far removed from bureaucracy and 'the grindset' as possible – and that doesn't make me lazy. It is okay to dream of a peaceful life as opposed to a busy life. It's okay to not be a model employee, it's okay to not enjoy going to work, and to prioritize the time you have to rest and do things you actually enjoy.

If you feel guilty in a moment of stillness, remind yourself that taking care of your mental health is productive. Getting rest is productive – prioritizing wellness is productive. You don't need to compare your productivity to other people's, because we all have different values and ideas of how a productive day is structured. It's time to redefine productivity to mean 'what makes you feel like you had a good and eventful day'.

You are not a machine put on this world to work until you drop, you are a person with needs and dreams that go beyond just career, and your productivity does not define your worth.

WAYS TO STOP PUTTING SO MUCH PRESSURE ON YOURSELF

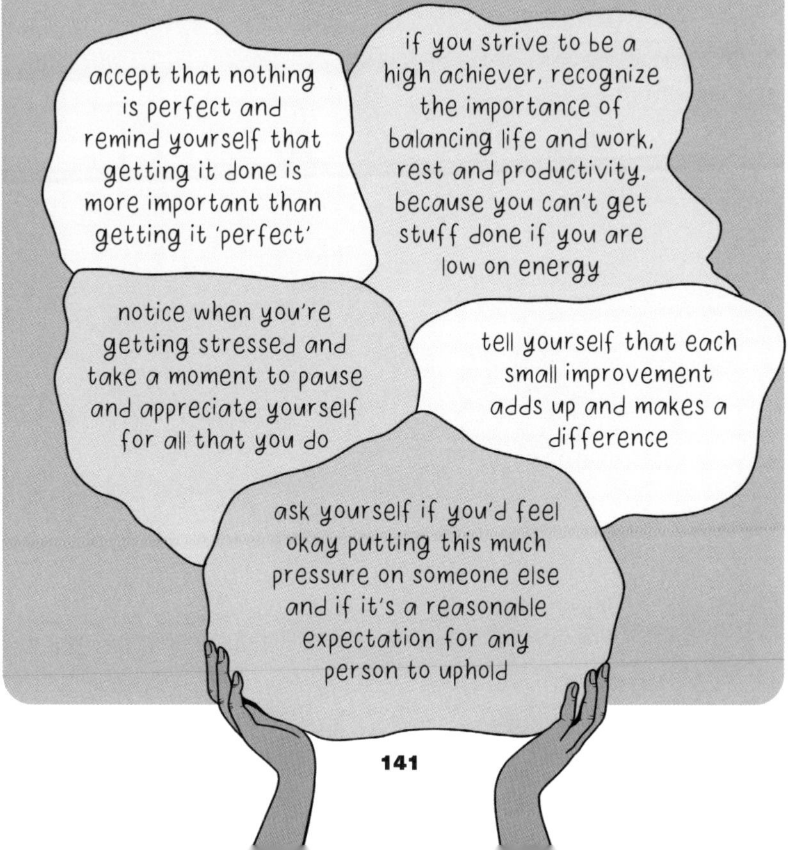
accept that nothing is perfect and remind yourself that getting it done is more important than getting it 'perfect'
if you strive to be a high achiever, recognize the importance of balancing life and work, rest and productivity, because you can't get stuff done if you are low on energy
notice when you're getting stressed and take a moment to pause and appreciate yourself for all that you do
tell yourself that each small improvement adds up and makes a difference
ask yourself if you'd feel okay putting this much pressure on someone else and if it's a reasonable expectation for any person to uphold

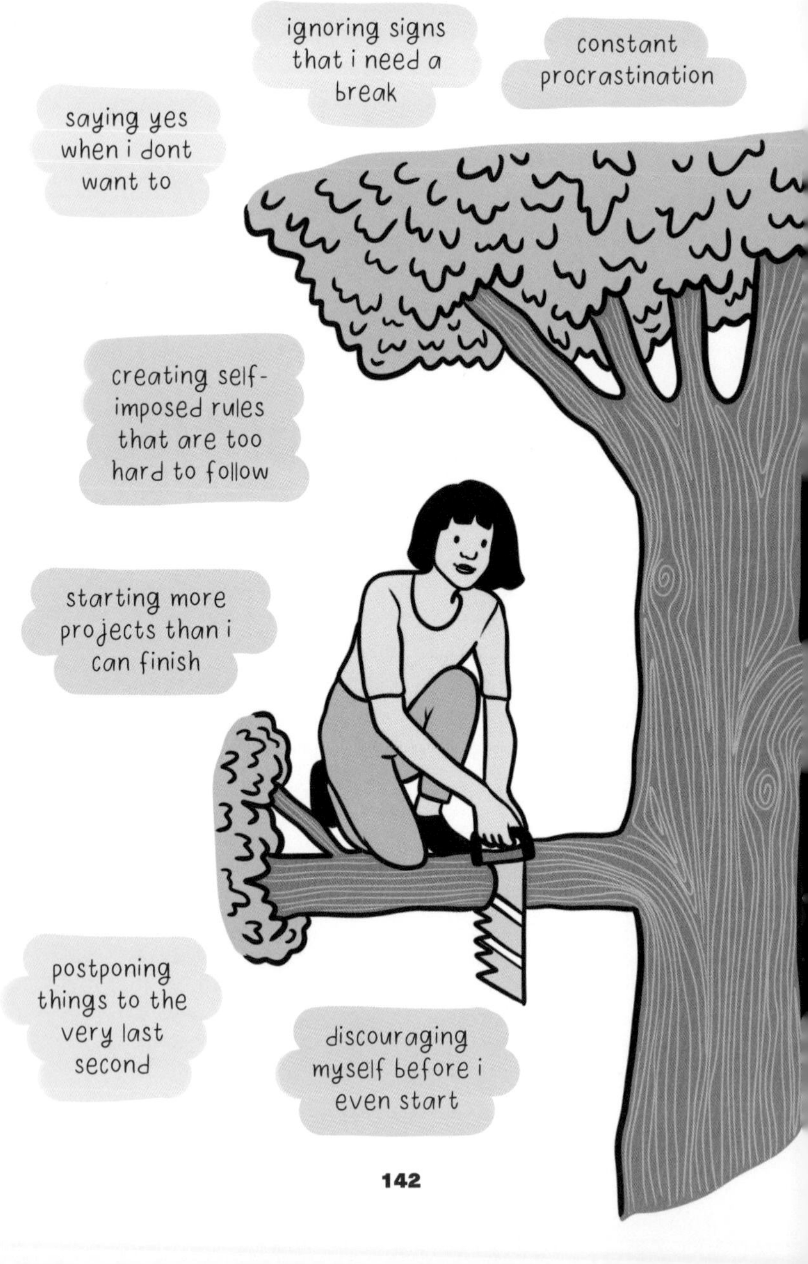
ignoring signs that i need a break
constant procrastination
saying yes when i dont want to
creating self-imposed rules that are too hard to follow
starting more projects than i can finish
postponing things to the very last second
discouraging myself before i even start

Am I self-sabotaging?

Self-sabotage and I have been well-acquainted for a long time. At first, I wouldn't quite recognize that I was doing it, but even when I did, I couldn't stop. It started with small things, like procrastinating with an essay until the very last day, or staying up too late the evening before an important day. On bad days it became skipping much-needed therapy, or spending too much money too early in the month, or saying, 'To hell with it', and giving up on something I worked a long time for. Needless to say, this did nothing for my mental state in the long-run.

not allowing myself things because i haven't 'earned it'

quitting when i run into an issue

overcomplicating solutions to small problems

Why do I self-sabotage, though? Shouldn't I be wanting to succeed, and shouldn't I be on my own side? It may be because, at times, I have struggled with low self-worth and I didn't believe I deserved to succeed. At other times, perhaps it's because I am seeking out simple pleasures, even when those pleasures are destructive, because happiness hasn't come easy. My ADHD also makes me feel bored easily, and so

I've done my fair share of pleasure-seeking to relieve the strain of under-stimulation. At other times, I indulge in self-sabotaging behaviour because the future is unsure, and as a last attempt to regain control I choose to give up, because failing because I decided to fail is easier than failing because I couldn't do it.

Whatever the reason, one of the easiest ways to figure out whether you're self-sabotaging is to ask yourself whether your current behaviours are in alignment with your goals and values. Sometimes we can feel stuck, demotivated to fulfil our own needs, and when life feels overwhelming it can be difficult to

SIGNS OF SELF-SABOTAGE

you don't set boundaries with others

you criticize yourself harshly

you don't ask for help or take necessary breaks

you set unrealistic goals and expectations

you feel stuck in self-destructive cycles

you feel like your life is chaotic and disorganized

you flee from negative emotions

you hold yourself back

you see the negative in every situation

recognize that. If we feel helpless, it can be hard to know if the patterns you have developed are actually serving you or not. If you're not sure, try asking yourself:

- Do I deny myself relaxation and simple joys only to overdo it later?
- Do I feel like I need better routines in daily life?
- Do I create self-imposed rules that trigger feelings of inadequacy?
- Do I ever self-generate stress, for example by biting off more than I can chew?

If you realize you're prone to self-sabotaging behaviours, it's time to figure out when you do it, so you can catch yourself next time. What areas of life do you sabotage, and what's happening right before you sabotage? What emotions do you experience when you feel the urge to sabotage? Do you ever do it without realizing it in the moment, and, if so, what are some clues leading up to it? It's important to be honest when examining our own responses to stress, feelings of inadequacy or lack of control. Self-sabotage can often stem from

negative thinking patterns, so once we address the part of us that tells us we don't deserve better, we can improve our mental health at the same time as we quash self-sabotage (see page 146).

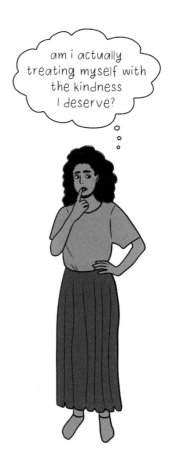

am i actually treating myself with the kindness I deserve?

STRATEGIES TO STOP
SELF-SABOTAGING

don't set goals for yourself that are too rigid or which lack clarity

identify what you truly want. are you self-sabotaging or is your gut telling you that this job, relationship, etc. isn't for you?

replace one self-sabotaging habit with a positive counter habit

practice positive self-talk as a way to combat your negative thoughts

think of ways to soothe yourself when you feel the urge to self-sabotage

reframe the way you look at failure and remember that it's a part of the human experience

ask yourself, if i was giving this task to someone else, would i be as harsh on them if they struggled with it?

ask a friend to help remind you of what you need to get done

reward yourself when you choose a healthy coping mechanism over self-sabotaging behaviours

get rid of things that trigger your self-sabotage

'I can't stop comparing myself to other people'

what if my life could be as easy as his?
i wish i could be as smart as she is

We all have things about ourselves that we wish were different, and we all sometimes see things in others that we wish we had. As children we start to notice differences between ourselves and others, but as we grow older these comparisons start to impact our self-esteem.

Life is full of moments where we get to observe the success of others. Maybe you're scrolling on Instagram one cold winter evening and see that your old friend moved to a luxury penthouse with the help of the generous salary they have. Perhaps you're having lunch with friends and one of them shows off a big engagement ring and talks about honeymoon plans. Or you have a sibling that you were compared with all your life and they're seemingly getting their life together, and you feel like you're always coming up short – and you

i wish i could be as confident as them

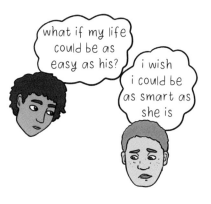

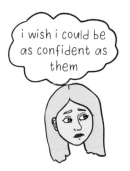

get that feeling. That icky bubbling of jealousy, followed by shame for not feeling happy enough for them, on top of feeling inadequate.

It's hard not to compare sometimes. Comparison reveals three things about ourselves: what we wish we had, what we are convinced we lack and what our view of success is. It can sometimes serve as a blueprint for positive change, if the comparison inspires us to seek opportunities and better ourselves in a healthy way. But, more often than not, comparison is a way we tear ourselves down. Seeing what others have, and what they're doing, can make us feel like what we have and do isn't enough.

Constant comparison is one of the fastest ways to obliterate our sense of self-worth, so it is important to catch ourselves doing it, and be gentle with ourselves.

The next time you find yourself feeling jealousy bubbling within, try this: get out a piece of paper, or open the notes app on your phone, and dig into that feeling. Analyze why it might be happening with the help of these questions:

- Can I reframe this jealousy into admiration? What do I like about this person that makes me feel this way, and can I try to appreciate them without pitting myself against them?
- Do I feel jealous because I am reminded of my own needs that are unmet? What are some ways I can ask for them to be met? Do I have any longings that are unaddressed?

i wish i had as many friends as him

i wish people respected me as easily as they respect him

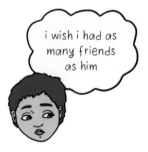

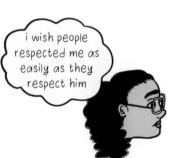

- Am I feeling jealousy because I fear I might be abandoned? What are some ways I can talk about that? What will it take for me to feel safer in my attachments with others?
- Is this jealousy my intuition trying to tell me that I'm not being appreciated or cared for in a way that makes me feel good and safe? Have my boundaries been respected?

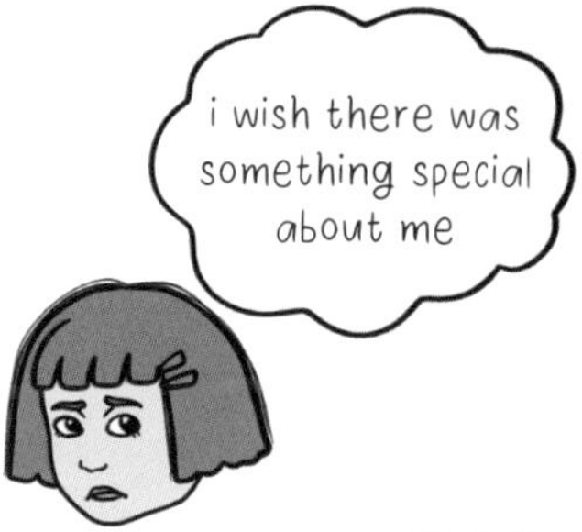
i wish there was something special about me

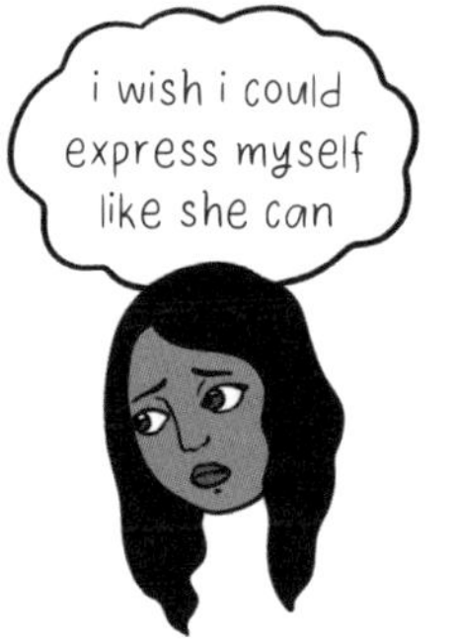
i wish i could express myself like she can

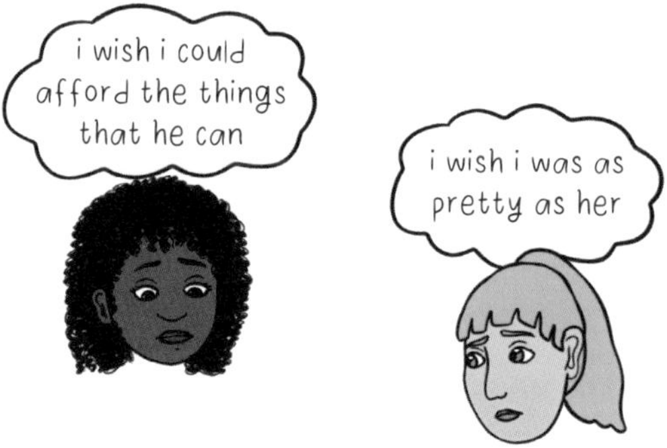
i wish i could afford the things that he can
i wish i was as pretty as her

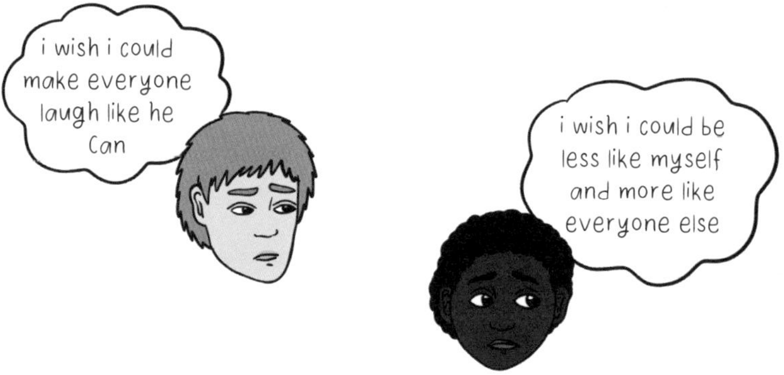
i wish i could make everyone laugh like he can
i wish i could be less like myself and more like everyone else

WAYS TO STOP COMPARING

keep a record of your achievements and celebrate them, no matter how big or small

recognize that even the person you're comparing yourself to has insecurities of their own

remind yourself that social media is full of posing, editing and people sharing their best moments. you don't see everything that goes wrong for someone on their feed

shift your focus to the things you're grateful for and the goals and dreams you want to achieve

remember just how special and unique you are and how there's nobody quite like you in this world

remember that we tend to compare the best of others to the worst of ourselves

talk to someone about it.
you might be surprised
how many people can
relate to this feeling

compliment yourself like you'd
compliment others, start
noticing and verbalizing your
best qualities

take a step back from
people and situations that
make you feel inferior,
and focus on self-care

give yourself credit for
how far you've come and
how much you have grown
throughout your life

Social media and loneliness

My first phone was a brick Nokia that I used for calls, the occasional text, and to play a pixelated game of snake. When Instagram first launched, my friends and I downloaded it and it felt fun and mindless; we posted silly pictures and got three likes on our posts, and it was only used to connect with close friends. Our feeds weren't full of influencers, photoshopped photos, brand deals and advertisements.

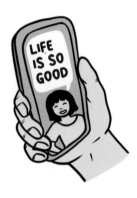

Social media looks different now and it's not designed with our long-term happiness in mind – quite the opposite. The way it's designed is reminiscent of a slot machine, but instead of pulling a lever we swipe up to refresh a page. Sometimes we are met with an exciting piece of media, which gives our brain a boost of dopamine. Dopamine is a way for the brain to let us know what's worth doing again and again. The unpredictability of this potential 'reward' keeps us coming back. And now a lot of apps have 'endless scrolling', which eats away at our time without us even realizing. Taking away those natural end points gives social media companies the opportunity to sell our attention to advertisers, but it can make us feel like we cannot step away and can even lead to addictions – a scary reality.

On top of this, seeing manipulated photos of 'ideal' bodies and luxurious lives can really mess with our self-esteem. Many studies show how a record number of teens feel dissatisfied with their bodies, and why wouldn't they when they're being constantly bombarded with this stuff? When I was a kid I would compare myself with the pretty girls in my grade. Now I have the opportunity to compare myself with photoshopped influencers, who themselves cannot even measure up to the ideal without posing, sucking in, and using Facetune.

But even if you manage to resist all of that, just seeing your friends enjoying life through carefully curated, beautiful pictures on your screen – while you're in bed, after a long and difficult day – can really make you feel like you're wasting your life watching others having fun. In short, it can make you feel lonely.

Once I was scrolling my phone, and I saw that my friends had all gathered to play boardgames, without inviting me, and I felt so excluded I called them on FaceTime in tears. They were confused and said, 'But you hate playing board games?' And I paused and said, 'Yeah, well, it would have been nice to be invited.' I probably wouldn't have gone, but somewhere in my mind I couldn't help but wonder if they were having more fun when I wasn't there. And if I hadn't seen it on social media, I would've just carried on having a relaxing day at home. Instead I had a big taste of loneliness and FOMO (Fear of Missing Out). My friends and I often joke lovingly about the severity of my FOMO, but I have realized that being alone, for me, is a huge trigger for feelings of worthlessness, and can put me at the centre of a downward spiral.

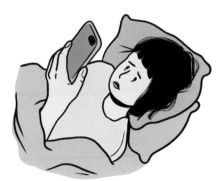

FOMO CAN FEEL LIKE

worrying that you
are missing out
on significant
fundamental human
experiences that
everyone else
'seems to have'

worrying that your
friends don't like
you any more when
they do things
without you
sometimes

feeling
regret when
you say no
to plans
because
you might
miss out on
something

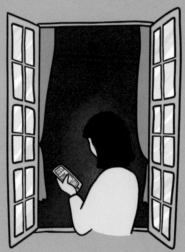

feeling insecure
when you see
people having
fun without
you there

saying yes to things
you don't want to do
because it feels
worse not to be
included

constantly focusing
on things you lack,
rather than the
things you have

feeling 'out of the
look' in life

I feel most like myself when I'm around others, and sometimes I feel proudest of myself when I get praise in the forms of comments and likes on social media, because of the immediate reward it feeds my brain. Coming to this realization really unsettled me, so to combat feeling that way, I wrote a list of things I needed to remember in those moments:

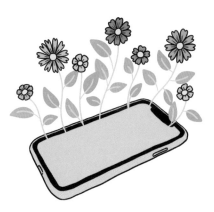

- I need a big step back from social media.
- I need to think of fulfilling things to do when I'm alone.
- I need to work on internal validation over external praise.
- I need to curate a more healthy social media experience.
- I need to trust that my friends like me, even when I'm not there.
- I have worked hard to find contentment in solitude.

Sometimes I say 'no' to seeing friends so I can practice being by myself, without worrying about what I might be missing. I take pictures to print out and save as memories, without having to put them on social media for everyone to see. I'm trying my best to see social media as an opportunity to catch up with friends, as opposed to using it as a highlight reel for accomplishments and my best selfies.

Negative feelings can act as cues that something needs changing. If you find yourself feeling empty or lonely after being on social media, it might be time to change the way you consume it. Reminding yourself that social media is often curated can help with comparison, and limiting your time online can remind you of the things that matter to you outside of it. If you are worried about social media dependency, you're not alone; see the 'further resources' on page 190 to learn more.

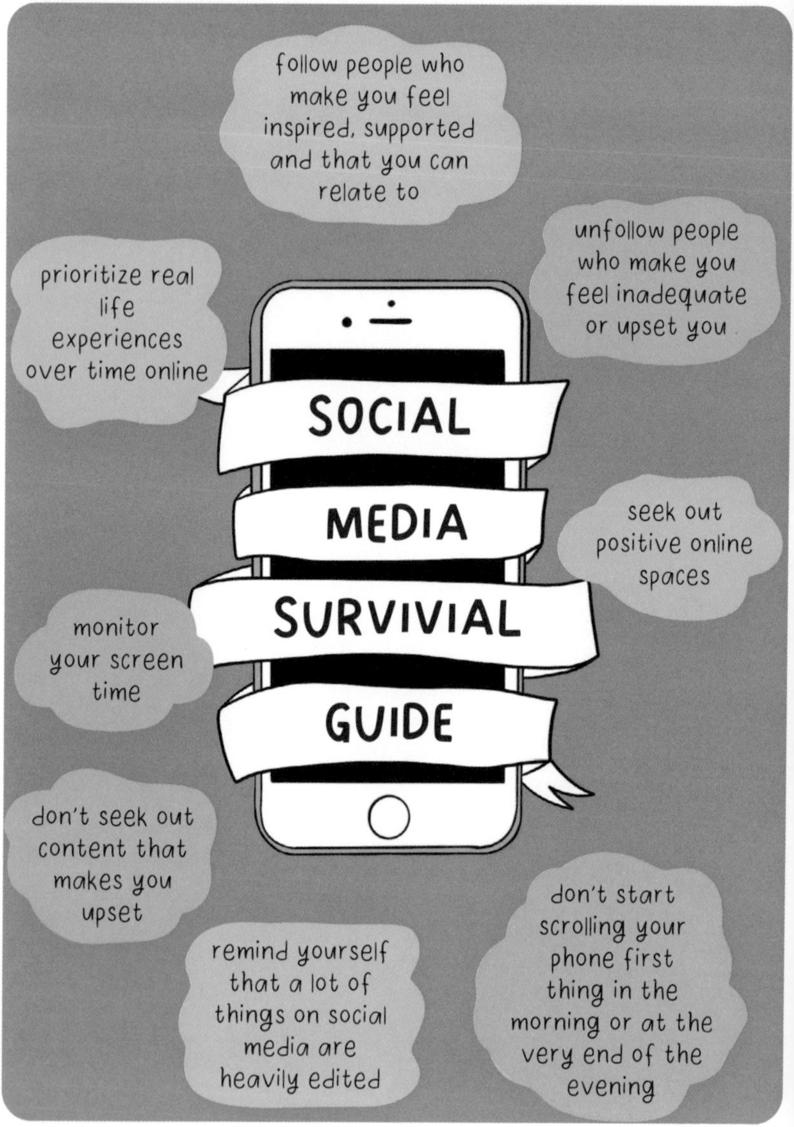
SOCIAL MEDIA SURVIVIAL GUIDE
follow people who make you feel inspired, supported and that you can relate to
unfollow people who make you feel inadequate or upset you
prioritize real life experiences over time online
seek out positive online spaces
monitor your screen time
don't seek out content that makes you upset
remind yourself that a lot of things on social media are heavily edited
don't start scrolling your phone first thing in the morning or at the very end of the evening

Relationships and mental illness

A good relationship can help improve our mental health. The support we receive from positive platonic, familial or romantic relationships can give us security and feelings of belonging.

Unstable or painful relationships, however, can make mental illness worse, and your mental health can have an effect on the dynamics of any relationship.

At seventeen, I met a special someone; he was visiting from America, doing an exchange year, and for the first time in my life, I felt a little twinge of romantic

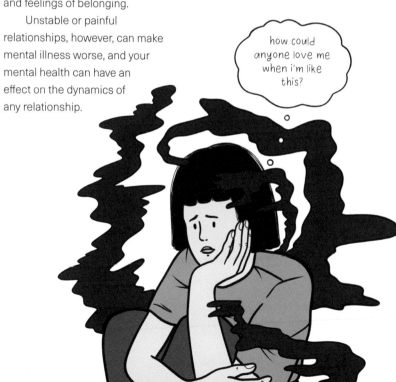

how could anyone love me when i'm like this?

DATING WITH MENTAL ILLNESS

if you want a long-term relationship, be open and honest with what you're going through

encourage your partner to get informed on what you're going through so they can better understand how to best support you on your journey

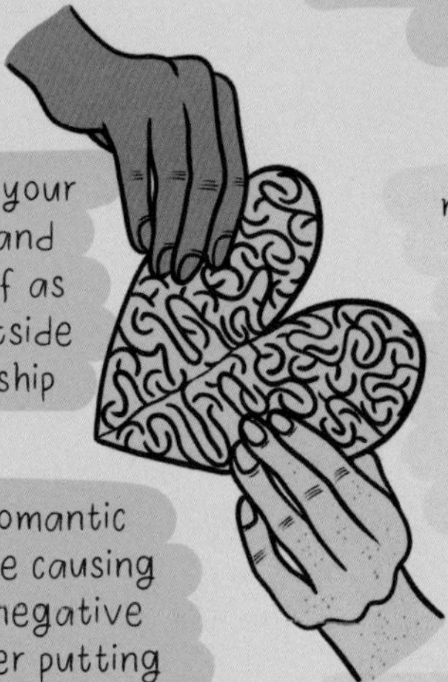

keep prioritising your mental health and work on yourself as an individual outside of the relationship

make sure you have several people who can help you in different ways, so that your partner doesn't have to be your sole support

if dating or romantic relationships are causing you stress or negative feelings, consider putting those things on hold until you feel ready

remember that mental illness does not make you incapable or undeserving of love and meaningful relationships

with mental illness, you and your partner have to accept that it might not always be an equal give and take. sometimes you don't have much energy to give desire growing in my heart. When his exchange year was coming to an end, I was devastated. He wanted to stay in Sweden but he didn't have anywhere to stay – I was surprised when my mother suggested he just stay with us. And he did: we lived in my childhood home until we got our own place.

Loving someone really is special: a love that makes you feel like everything had been leading up to that first meeting, a love that's a cushion against the hardness of the world, making it feel a lot more bearable.

I didn't know how mental illness and love would mix in my brain, but it turns out it can get quite intense. The serotonin that love gave me was addictive, and I would do anything to protect that love. I felt anxious, my self-esteem was low, and I would often wonder if my hypersensitivity and moods would push him away. Even in friendships, mental illness felt like a third wheel, a lone dark cloud in an otherwise blue sky, and it made it hard to be a good friend sometimes. It's tough to be there for others when you can barely keep yourself afloat, and in the give and take of relationships, mental illness can make you feel so empty – you reach inside but there's nothing to give your loved one who needs you.

I put a lot on my partner, because I was young and I had all these feelings, and someone who I felt I could finally share everything with. But the voice in the back of my head kept asking, 'How long can he deal with me?' If I'm exhausted by spending time alone with my thoughts, I wonder how exhausted he'd feel hearing about it. He never made me feel wrong or like a burden, but since I valued our relationship so much, I decided to actively work on maintaining a healthy relationship, and being a partner who could do an equal give and take.

People with mental illness are more likely to be victims of violence and abuse than the general public. Unfortunately, many people grow up without the luxury of having healthy relationships modelled to them as children, so some reach adulthood without a clear example of what healthy and supportive relationships should look and feel like.

This could make a person vulnerable and susceptible to finding themselves in toxic or abusive relationships as teens and adults. If we lack boundaries and self-respect, we run the risk of being taken advantage of.

Mental health conditions can be a hurdle in our relationships, and to overcome this, we need to build our relationship with ourselves, outside of our other connections. That's not to say that there isn't space to work together with friends, family and romantic partners, but a steady foundation with yourself is key. I don't believe you have to love yourself to be

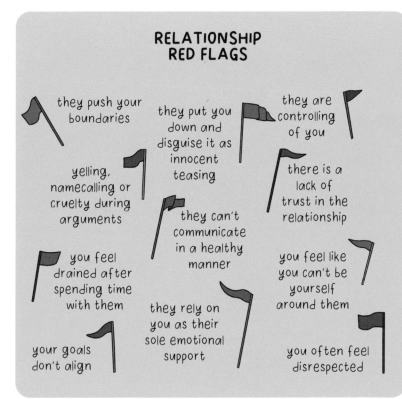

RELATIONSHIP RED FLAGS

- they push your boundaries
- they put you down and disguise it as innocent teasing
- they are controlling of you
- yelling, namecalling or cruelty during arguments
- there is a lack of trust in the relationship
- they can't communicate in a healthy manner
- you feel drained after spending time with them
- you feel like you can't be yourself around them
- they rely on you as their sole emotional support
- your goals don't align
- you often feel disrespected

able to love others. Self-love can be hard and complicated and take a long time to achieve, but it's an absolute necessity to be able to set boundaries, to view yourself as someone who deserves to be treated with kindness and respect, and to communicate your needs and wants – otherwise we might accept behaviours that are harmful to us and our mental health. People who won't treat you in a way that makes you feel safe and supported aren't people who deserve to be in your life.

RELATIONSHIP GREEN FLAGS

you feel heard, understood and supported

they are able to express their feelings in healthy ways

it feels easy to love them and be loved in return

you feel comfortable disagreeing with them

you share similar values and goals

you approach problems as a team

they are reliable and prioritize you

you grow as a couple as well as individuals

they make it clear that they love you

they respect your limits and boundaries

you have fun together

Grief and loss

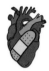

This chapter deals with experiences of grief and death. If this is too much right now, please skip ahead to page 168.

Out of all of life's difficult experiences, losing someone or something important to you has to be one of the hardest. Grief is the price we pay for love – mourning is love that has nowhere to go. And I haven't met a pain quite as severe as longing for someone who isn't here anymore. I managed to avoid loss until I was 20, when my grandpa passed from fast and aggressive pancreatic cancer. Being petrified of death and the very concept of mortality, his descent into illness felt like a blur. The only thing I remember vividly is seeing him, much frailer, sitting on his leather couch, listening to Bruce Springsteen singing 'I don't want to fade away' on his record player – and I wondered if he knew what the lyrics meant. The day he died I visited him at the hospital and I was inconsolable, because somehow I knew it would be the last time, but I didn't want to vocalize or think about that. He took his last breath three days before my birthday, which then felt bizarre and pointless to celebrate.

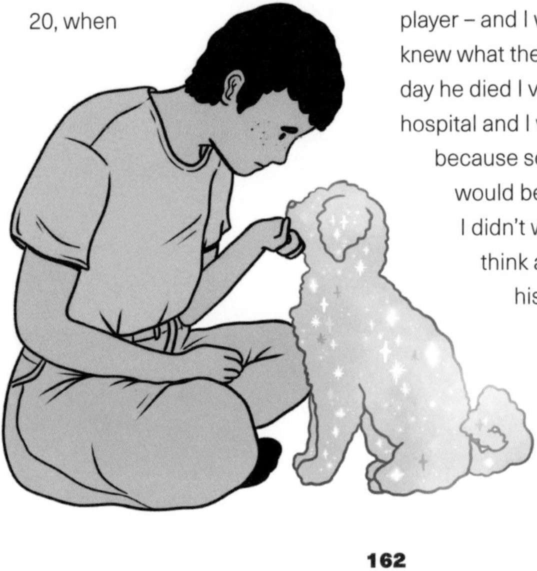

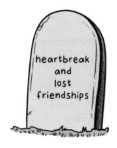

heartbreak and lost friendships

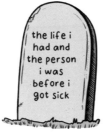

the life i had and the person i was before i got sick

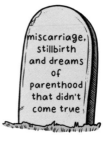

miscarriage, stillbirth and dreams of parenthood that didn't come true

I didn't expect the reaction I had to grief. I withdrew into myself, like a hermit crab contracting into its hard shell. I didn't want to share my grief with anyone, or partake in ceremonies of shared mourning. My own grief was painful, but seeing the grief of my family made it ten times harder. It suffocated me, it sat like a big black hole in every room, a collective weight none of us could properly put down. One person's absence changed everything, forever. But as painful as my grief was, it was also sacred – it was a force that could keep me tethered to someone who had gone beyond our realm – a reminder of him. Grief is so complex, because death is so incomprehensible to us.

Grieving the loss of my grandpa made me realize that I had mourned before, many times. Because grief isn't only felt when someone we love dies, it also presents itself when a relationship goes away, or when we lose something that was important to us.

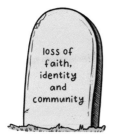

loss of faith, identity and community

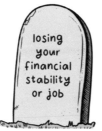

losing your financial stability or job

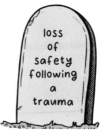

loss of safety following a trauma

There is no right or wrong way to grieve. It's okay if you cry every day, it's okay if you don't cry at all. It's fine to want to talk about it often, or to process it by yourself. I would wonder, 'When will this stop hurting so much, when will the grief go away?' But after time I realized that grief doesn't really go away. You don't just get over losing someone, and that loss will make itself known when something reminds us of them: when their birthday is coming up, when something new happens in life and we wish we could tell them all about it. Just like we cannot bring someone back to us, we cannot erase grief completely. But as the days become weeks and months and years, we slowly get used to the absence. Life continues to expand, and one day we think of them, and notice that the reminder doesn't feel like a punch in the gut, but like a warm, distant memory. We learn to honour our grief, and to live alongside it.

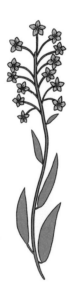

But in the meantime, while the grief is fresh and all-consuming, it's important to tend to our emotional health. Mourning is a natural process, but there are ways to help ourselves along the way, to make it a little easier to get through the initial stages where it feels the most difficult (see page 167 for my suggestions). Although grief can be absolutely excruciating, there is a difference between grief and depression, and if your grief continues to interfere with your sleep and appetite, if it makes you feel like your own life is shrinking, it might be time to speak to a professional.

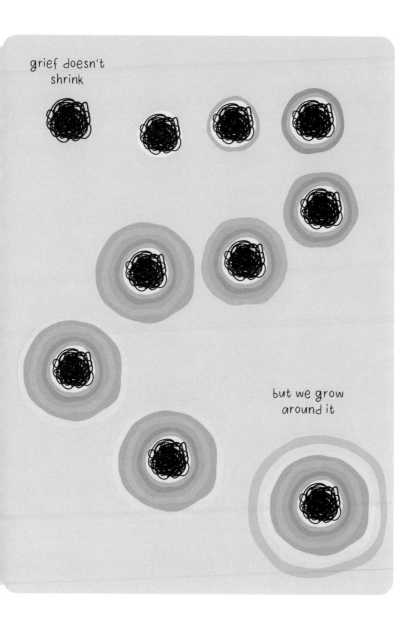

grief doesn't
shrink

but we grow
around it

I think it's important to let yourself be devastated in the face of loss, as grief is natural. There are so many ways that grief can present itself, and that's okay. From having experienced grief and witnessing it in other people, I know how deeply it hurts, and how it feels like nothing will ever be the same – and it won't be the same, but it will get easier. As time passes, and life continues bringing new experiences, it won't be as insurmountable. Grief can be a long process that never ends completely, but, as we continue on, time will help us heal. Self-care is an important part of healing through grief, so building those tools and implementing them into daily life can act like a life-vest. Making time to be around others, going outside, sitting with your feelings mindfully, wrapping yourself up on chilly evenings, soothing yourself with sounds or smells or tastes: this is how we can build an arsenal of ways to make the days feel easier. And as we do start to feel a bit better and like ourselves again, remember that it doesn't mean you are betraying or undermining the love you had for who or what you lost. It's easy to feel a twinge of guilt when you think about your loss less and less often, so be kind to yourself through all the feelings grief might bring. There is no wrong way to feel or process, or remember.

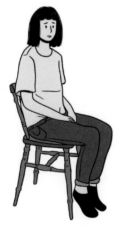
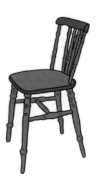

COPING WITH GRIEF

prioritze your sleep, eating and emotional needs

take active steps to treasure and celebrate the lives of and bonds with your loved ones

try to keep a routine to make the days fuller

allow yourself time and space to feel and express your emotions

remember that no feelings are wrong

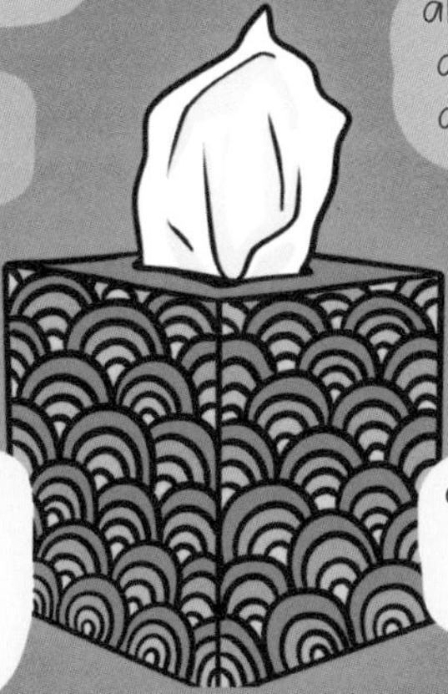

don't be scared to accept or ask for help with practical tasks if you feel overwhelmed

avoid making big decisions in the midst of grief

consider starting a new tradition to celebrate the one you lost and to connect with their memory

talk about your grief with someone you trust, or keep a journal for processing your thoughts throughout the mourning process

Keep going!

As I entered my twenties, I would often stop to think, 'When will things just go my way? When will all these difficulties end? Why do things go wrong so often?' But the truth is, life will always have difficulties, there will be days where it feels like everything goes wrong all at once. One of the biggest challenges us humans face is learning to be okay with uncertainty and roadblocks. When you're actively working on healing your mental health, even the smallest of inconveniences can turn a good day into a battle.

A big part of improving your mental health is getting to know your needs, and discovering ways to comfort yourself. Part of this is collecting the mental tools to build stress tolerance, and creating a layer of padding between you and stress by designating time for activities that lift your spirit. Divide problems into things that can be controlled, improved or solved, and things that we need to accept as inevitable, but which you can approach in different ways to give yourself solace and encouragement.

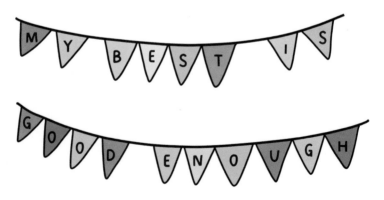

REMEMBER ...

Practice managing your stress

•

Take time to relax

•

Address any self-sabotage

•

Everyone's journey is individual,
comparisons aren't helpful

•

Use social media
with kindness and care

•

Healthy relationships are
compatible with your mental health

•

Grief is a process you will go
through

Chapter 5

YOU CAN THRIVE, NOT JUST SURVIVE

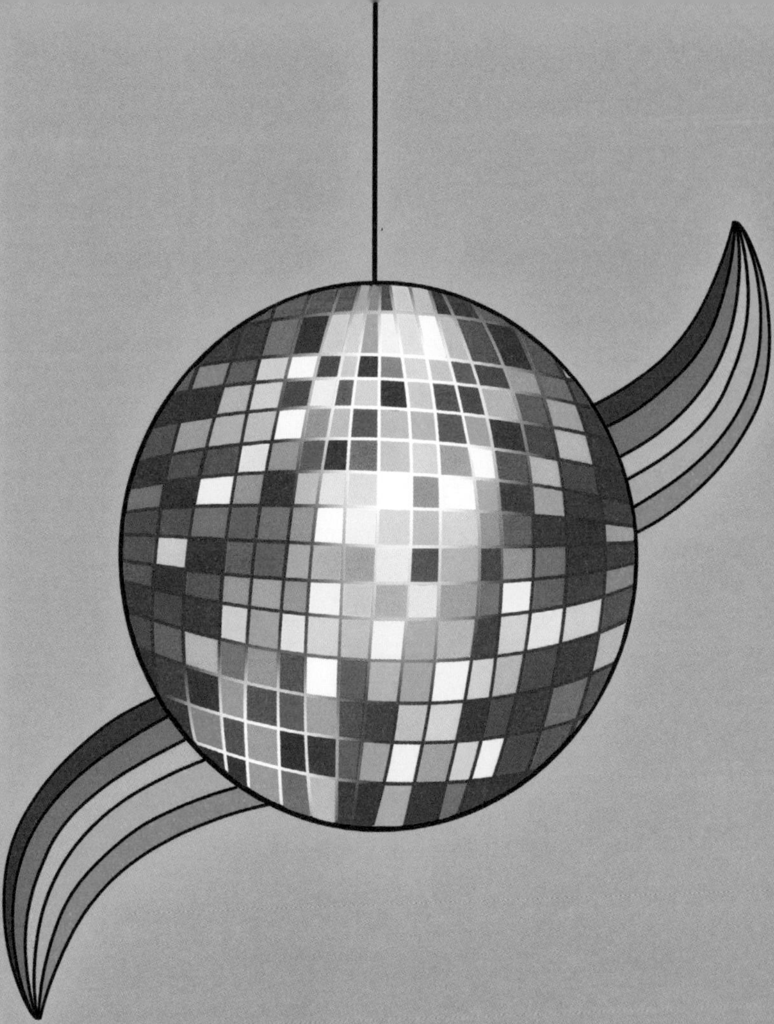

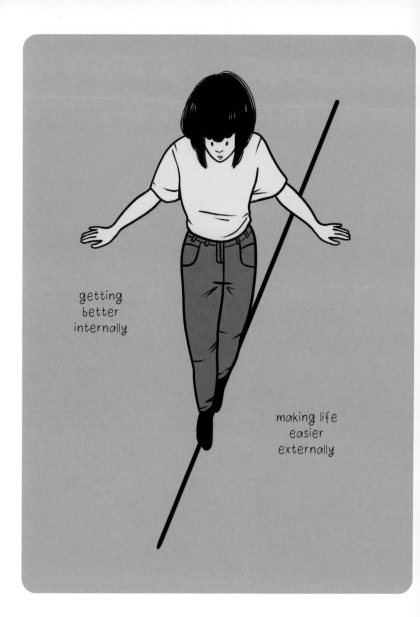

getting
better
internally

making life
easier
externally

Making life work for you

When you feel stuck in survival mode, the idea that you'll one day find contentment may seem so far away that it's impossible to imagine. It took me seeing and meeting other people with similar challenges, who found ways to thrive, for me to be motivated to turn my life around. Life will always bring new challenges, but when we take the time to get to know other people's struggles, it's evident that we all face hardships, and it's up to us all as individuals to ask: 'How can I make life work better for me? How can I honour my needs each day?'

One of my biggest gripes with mental health care is that, in my experience, the focus is often solely on treating symptoms, usually with medications and talk therapy, but we rarely talk about how to make life more liveable. I did need meds to feel better,

but I never felt like my care was personalized to my individual needs. I was told my mental illness stemmed from faulty chemistry in my brain, but daily stressors and unresolved trauma were making it worse than it had to be.

I had lots of questions. Am I living my life according to my values? Do I see a lack of meaning, like something is missing from life? Am I actually prioritizing mental health, and is it even possible in our modern world to put our mental health needs before our many responsibilities?

Thinking back to my childhood with undiagnosed learning disabilities, and the pain of being neurodivergent without knowing it for a long time, I realise now that I'd had to adapt. Since my problems remained unnoticed and unaddressed for so long, I coped by coming up with my own ways of doing things. In first grade, I made friends with a Polish girl who didn't speak Swedish yet, and it was easier to 'talk' to her than to my Swedish-speaking peers. I brought stuffed animals to school to soothe my nervousness way beyond a 'normal' age, and I had a designated hiding spot at school where I would go and have a good cry when things overwhelmed me. My then-undiagnosed dyscalculia made maths class particularly hellish (I have severe maths anxiety to this day) and I had to think of ways to count that made sense to me. And now, as an adult, I am still figuring out ways to work with my brain, not against it.

When you understand yourself, you can start thinking of ways to work around things you find difficult and help yourself thrive. You don't have to do things the way others do, and you don't have to do them perfectly. You can find your own values and beliefs to live by, according to what speaks to you, and you can build in activities that you know lift you up. For example, I love listening to educational podcasts when I do boring household tasks, because then it feels like I'm learning something instead of being stuck in a loop of chores. After a while, it feels like I'm on autopilot, and my body is doing its own thing while my mind is being nourished with interesting facts. ADHD has made it challenging for me to properly plan and organize, so I've come up with various little 'ADHD-hacks' that make it easier for me to get stuff done.

When I do prep for the coming day, I always say, 'Future Matilda is gonna be so pumped that past Matilda did this for her!' Everything I bring into my house gets a designated 'home' so I can keep track of my things. My daily routine has been carefully crafted over months of trial and error to suit my specific needs and abilities. To make your own supportive routine, I suggest writing down your most common problems, and with the help of a trusted friend or some Googling, identifying ways to work around them – ways that make sense to you, and that are actually doable.

PROBLEM	SOLUTION
i can never find my wallet	get a brightly coloured wallet
i can't do my dishes when i'm depressed	eat from paper plates when you're depressed
i can't keep track of my tasks	set reminders on your phone and write tasks down on post it notes
i isolate and neglect my relationships when i'm down	plan social interaction into your weekly schedule
i forget to take my meds	stick your meds on the inside of the front door at eye level
the house is so messy and i don't know where to start	set a timer for fifteen mins, put on music and do as much as you can
i can't bring myself to do tedious tasks	have a friend act as 'body double' to help you and do it together
i procrastinate until the last minute	set a mock deadline before your actual deadline and follow that instead

A big part of making life feel more manageable is getting to know ourselves and our needs. One of the risks of poor mental health is developing an unstable sense of self. Becoming better doesn't have to mean changing every part of yourself – we all have different strengths and challenges – it's about finding ways to work with your strengths and around your challenges.

This is where learning to practice self-leadership can really help. Self-leadership is a way to help you achieve goals and make life easier by identifying who you are in the present moment: your traits, values and interests. Based on all those parts of yourself, you can work out your personal goals and how you can best motivate yourself, using your strengths to get there.

Some manageable steps to develop your self-leadership skills are:

- Identifying achievable personal goals, whether it's doing the dishes every day or finding a job that fulfils you more.
- Monitoring your progress

towards those goals, and celebrate wins big or small.

- Thinking about your strengths and how you can use them to further your goals.
- Writing down three new habits you'd like to incorporate into your life, such as practicing setting boundaries, or trying out a new organization tool to keep track of important things.
- Thinking about what triggers you to give up when it gets tough, and ask yourself how you can comfort yourself when faced with challenges.

Self-leadership means you are leading yourself, not looking to someone else to lead you. By creating habits that make it easier to get motivated and inspired, as well as finding ways to keep relatively organized that actually work for you, you can become your own champion. Sometimes it's good to get creative and embrace unconventional ways to work around challenges, especially when your mental health is in a fragile place.

I love self-leadership because it invites you to work on that growth mindset we discussed earlier; it gives you the freedom to define what matters to you, and how you can take care of your individual needs. When I was a teenager and was stuck in my fixed mindset, I gave up before attempting something new if I wasn't sure I'd be good at it. Because if I failed, I felt like I would lose control and might look incompetent. Now that I work daily to strengthen my growth mindset, I find control in allowing myself to try new things without expectation, finding bravery and empowerment in learning through trial and error. When you see failure as a guide for improvement, that is where you can find confidence to self-lead. To look to yourself as a safe person in your life, who will be there to cheer you on.

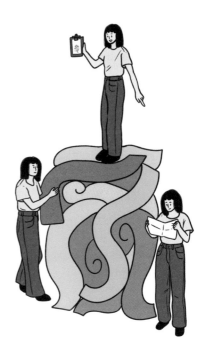

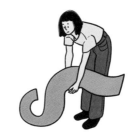

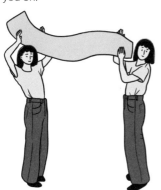

How I worry less

Unchecked worries are like snowflakes that can build up into heavy piles of snow if we leave them unaddressed. Everybody worries at times, but this can quickly manifest into physical stress and anxiety if we don't give ourselves time to process and challenge our worries.

Anxiety can make the most minor inconveniences feel like huge, imminent catastrophes. My anxiety has this funny way of making me feel like I'm about to die, and feeling like you're about to die tends to make you more anxious, so I get stuck in the most awful loop.

I had a lot of health anxiety as a teenager. And the more I worried, the worse it got. Until one moment where I got so sick of being scared, I just said: 'If I die, I die, and this is not my problem anymore.'

And it might sound harsh, but it worked. Death was my biggest fear, but the way my mind was scaring itself was worse. I reached this radical acceptance, that even if the worst case scenario happened, if I actually died, it's not like I could do anything about it. I would just die, like everyone does at some point, and the world would continue spinning. Me worrying about it was just making my suffering

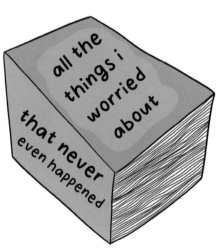

all the things i worried about that never even happened

worse, and every time I worried about death, I wasted time.

Am I going to worry about stuff that I can't even control until I actually die? Hell no. And why should I be so scared of death when it's as natural as birth, and when I don't even know what death is like? Why worry when I can't control the outcome? Why be scared when I can be curious instead?

You do yourself a huge disservice when you entertain all those pesky 'what ifs'. You prolong your suffering when you ruminate over things out of your control. Embracing even the worst outcome – practising radical acceptance – can help put a stop to that.

Another great antidote to my worrying was learning about distress tolerance. Distress tolerance is how we live though a moment of high-stress without making it worse or harder on ourselves. We don't always have control of situations, but we can learn how to better control our reactions during difficult moments. I can't avoid all stress in life, but I can improve the way I react to it. By building my distress tolerance with the coping tools I've collected, I am better adapted to handle the inevitable moments of stress and worry.

When I'm distressed, I like to take a couple of physical steps back, signalling to my brain that I am stepping away from the situation. And from where I now stand, I can observe. Observe the sensations in my body – where does the stress sit, what is going through my mind? After that, I shift my attention to my surroundings. Is there an actual danger? Is there a safe person nearby? A comfort object? Is it cloudy outside? Once I have observed, I try to think of a way to proceed mindfully. Should I get some air? Do I need to shake it off for a bit? Run in place? My favourite thing to do then is to retreat to the shower. I'll stand under the water, change it from hot to cold and just feel the sensations, gaining control of the way my body feels. I like to visualize the water rinsing my stress off, flowing into the drain and far away from me. Wrapping myself in a warm towel and breathing deeply, I can then say to myself, 'I got through that, the worst is over – I am safe even in moments where I feel extremely stressed.'

I have also started assigning my worries for my future self. If I am faced with a big worry and start to feel all that stress and fear creep up, I take a few deep breaths and tell myself that future Matilda can deal with this later. Present Matilda is too fragile and stressed to deal with this now, and since she's feeling helpless, she's not even up to worrying about this now. I put trust in my future self, that she will be able to handle it if she needs to. And usually, everything turns out just fine.

this is really stressing me out, i'm worried about the outcome of this
this seems like a problem for future Matilda. i'm just gonna put this aside and let her deal with it if it gets to that point!

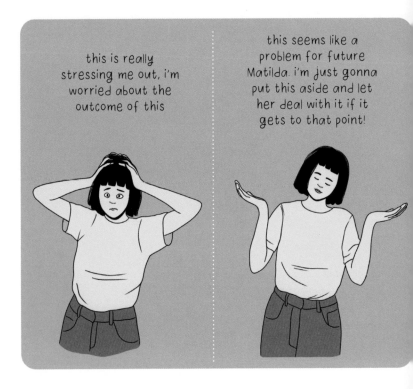

COPING
STATEMENTS

i've made it through this before

i am going to let this feeling slowly pass

some days are harder than others

i don't feel good so i'm gonna be extra nice
to myself

today was hard so i'm going to think of
ways to make tomorrow easier

i have yet to face a moment I couldn't make
it through

i can't change or control everything

my worst moments do not define me

pain is an inevitable part of life

i don't like this but i am able to adapt

Things to let go of

Things changing or going away has always been deeply troubling to me, as someone who feels her safest when life goes according to plan.

I think it's easy to romanticize the past, because the pain we feel now seems more real and urgent than the pain we felt in times past. Even if we know that, logically, moving on and putting things behind us is good, our emotional brain feels differently. If we lose a friend, for example, the love we feel for them doesn't go away just because they aren't in our life anymore. Letting go is especially painful when it's not up to us, when it's out of our control.

Moving on is essential for learning to live in the moment. The past cannot be changed: ruminating stops us from creating positive change in the now. I figured out a strategy I could use when I struggle to let go or move past something. For letting go, I try to think of something to add to my life to replace what I've lost.

Can I cultivate what I'm missing in another way? Am I longing for an apology that's not going to come? Do I need to give myself forgiveness for things I did wrong when I didn't know better? Do I need to cry it out or write it out? Sometimes I don't have any clear answers to these questions, and in those moments, I have some other tricks.

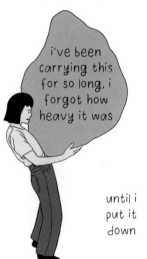

i've been carrying this for so long, i forgot how heavy it was

until i put it down

TIPS FOR HOW TO LET GO

remind yourself that things don't have to be permanent to matter or provide meaning in your life

give yourself time to grieve the loss and be gentle with yourself along the way

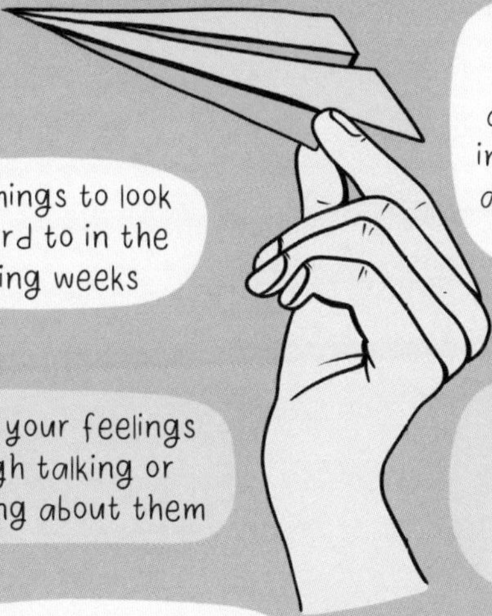

bring back focus to yourself. sit down and think of ways to improve your daily life and the moments you spend alone

plan things to look forward to in the coming weeks

express your feelings through talking or journaling about them

try to reflect realistically. it can be easy to idealize relationships after they've ended

create physical distance between you and the thing you're letting go of to make the transition easier

take yourself on a date to celebrate yourself

imagine yourself entering a new chapter of life and think of the possibilities of new beginnings

Look for
the silver linings

I resisted gratitude for a long time. Even though I had plenty to be thankful for – a loving family, financial stability – I didn't have the mental bandwidth to enjoy my privileges. Mental illness tends to sully even the brightest parts of our lives, it puts negativity at the front and centre. Happy people can be off-putting when you struggle to remember the last time you felt true joy or contentment. But gratitude is important, especially when life feels difficult, because reminding yourself of all the good can make the bad seem less heavy or prevalent. Gratitude doesn't mean ignoring the things that feel wrong or difficult, but it gives you space to appreciate what's good, even the little things. It plants little seeds of joy in the mundane.

Do you feel enough gratitude towards your life? You can measure this by asking yourself questions, like:

- When I look at the world, can I identify things I'm grateful for?
- Do I have frequent moments where I appreciate something?
- If I listed out things to be grateful for, would it be a long list?
- Can I find appreciation for little things in life?
- Does my appreciation for life grow bigger as I grow older?

If you answered no to a lot of the questions, take it as a sign to cultivate more gratitude in life. Your life doesn't have to be perfect or even easy to learn to practice gratitude. In fact, the act of giving thanks can make life feel fuller and more meaningful, which can improve our overall mood and outlook on life.

Gratitude can start with mindfulness. Simply observe your present moment: look around you. Feel yourself in your body – it has

SILVER LININGS OF MY MENTAL ILLNESS

i am very empathic to and supportive of other people's mental health troubles

i have connected with other people who relate to my struggles and understand what i'm going through

mental illness made me seek out and learn lots of information on how to get better, that i can use and share with others

sharing my story has helped other people feel validated and less alone and it has helped me assign meaning to my pain

i am much stronger now because of what i've dealt with, and i feel better equipped to handle tough times

having been incredibly low, i have found deep appreciation for moments of joy and will celebrate at every opportunity

my friends feel comfortable opening up to me about their own problems because i am open with mine taken you places, kept you warm, protected and alive. Look outside: see the grass and the sky and the clouds. Hear the sounds of other people living their lives. Think of how wild it is that our sun is at the perfect distance to provide us life, how cosmically lucky we are to live on this earth. And then, take a moment to savour thankfulness. Imagine your brain absorbing the good feelings, nourishing yourself.

Create a routine and habit around gratitude; you could set an alarm on your phone and, when it goes off, think of three things

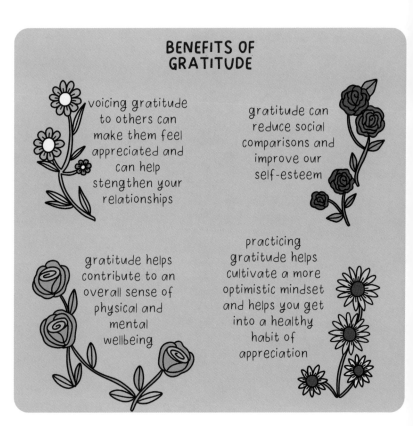

BENEFITS OF GRATITUDE

voicing gratitude to others can make them feel appreciated and can help stengthen your relationships

gratitude can reduce social comparisons and improve our self-esteem

gratitude helps contribute to an overall sense of physical and mental wellbeing

practicing gratitude helps cultivate a more optimistic mindset and helps you get into a healthy habit of appreciation you are grateful for. Voice your gratitude to others. When you feel appreciation for someone, tell them. When you eat a good meal, say out loud how good it is. Write a thank-you note to yourself for getting through so much. You don't have to believe that everything has a silver lining, because sometimes, things just hurt. There's no reason to force gratitude; instead, we can find gratitude in what helped us through – in our own resilience.

THINGS I'M THANKFUL FOR

- my ability to love other people
- the joy of finding a really good song
- when my indoor plants grow new leaves or flowers
- sleeping in freshly washed sheets after a shower
- freshly baked bread
- moments of uninterrupted belly laughs
- when i try a new baking recipe and it comes out just right
- when the weather gets warm enough to take the bike out
- when my grocery store buys in a new vegan ice cream flavour
- candid photos of good memories
- finding a good deal at the thrift store

My message to you

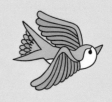

Healing is a lifelong journey, because as we grow and change, so do our needs and the challenges we face. As we get to know ourselves, we can discover more ways to navigate our unique paths. Thriving as you are doesn't mean getting things perfect, but learning to find joy in the ebbs and flows of life. There is nothing wrong with meeting yourself where you are, even if you aren't happy with where that might be at the moment.

It's never too late, or the wrong time, to look for things that make you happy, or to start implementing healthier habits to cultivate better mental health. Sometimes life feels full of things beyond our control, and it's demotivating and scary – but remember that regaining some of that control starts with making choices to prioritize yourself. The times where healing feels the hardest are often the times we need this the most, which is why it's important to not give up hope, and remind yourself that you deserve to take the time to do the work.

When writing this book, I had to remember a lot on the journey I have taken, from a scared child to suicidal tween to a desperate teenager, to a 24-year-old woman who keeps a strong hold on hope, believes in her own resilience, and respects herself enough to honour her needs. Going from wondering

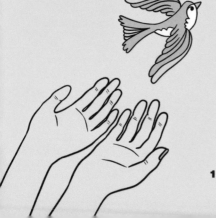

how to survive to the next day, to looking forward to the promise of tomorrow was once unfathomable, but now it's reality. A change that happened so incrementally, I didn't notice until I reflected back on it. All because of little steps every day, all the tips in these pages, resulting in a life I don't feel trapped in anymore, but which I am grateful to have – even with my mental health challenges.

We may have reached the end of this book, but not the end of our collective journeys. I hope you came away from this experience with some new understanding and new things to try, and permission to heal in ways that feel supportive to you. I hope that you feel validated. In a world where the stigma of mental illness and any mental struggle constricts us, prioritizing your mental health is an act of bravery. I hope you feel inspired to be kinder to yourself – to meet yourself where you are – and that you are hungry to learn more about mental health and yourself – because knowledge is empowering. When we give space to understand ourselves, forgive ourselves and practice kindness to ourselves, that is when we can start the journey towards feeling better.

Today is a perfect day to take the first step – to schedule a meaningful act of self-care in your daily calendar, to practice new coping skills, to find gratitude in something you've never noticed before. To book that doctor's appointment, or to reach out to someone safe. To check in with someone you love who you've recognized in these pages. To make progress at your own pace, with patience and forgiveness and hope, because you are worth it, and you always were.

As you continue your own journey, reflect on the changes you wish for, the needs you long to fulfil, and be open to trying whatever you feel might help. Build your mental health toolkit, define what joy or peace or motivation or hope looks like to you, try ways to cope and soothe and breathe and rewire your thoughts. Our brains are so adaptable, and there's a lot of empowerment to be found in that fact. And give yourself a big pat on the back, a warm hug and heartfelt praise for coming this far already.

USEFUL RESOURCES

Organizations for support
National Alliance on Mental
    Illness (NAMI)
verywellmind.com
Mind.org
National Eating Disorder
    Association (NEDA)
Rape Abuse and Incest National
    Network (RAINN)

Free worksheets
psychologytools.com
getselfhelp.co.uk
thinkcbt.com

Finding a therapist/someone to talk to
internationaltherapistdirectory.com
therapytribe.com
7cups.com
wellnite.com

BIPOC and LGBTQIA+
ayanatherapy.com
therapyforblackgirls.com
Shine (wellness app)
inclusivetherapists.com
thementalhealthcoalition.org
pridecounseling.com
thetrevorproject.org
translifeline.org

Free apps
MindShift (CBT exercises)
Daylio (Mood tracker)
BellyBio (neurofeedback for
    breathing)
Bearable (symptom tracker)
PTSD Coach
Mediotopia (mindfullness)

My favourite mental health Instagram communities
@crazyheadcomics
@drjulie
@anxiousblackgirlcomics
@doodledwellness
@selfcarespotlight
@hellomynameiswednesday
@thefriendineverwanted
@makedaisychains
@gmf.designs
@thepsychologymum
@minaa_b
@theburntoutbrain
@thatgoodgrief

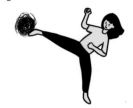

ACKNOWLEDGEMENTS

Boundless thanks and gratitude to my family and relatives, especially mom and dad for your gentle, encouraging parenting. For teaching me that no dream is too big or unrealistic to chase after. I never had to wonder if I was making you proud, because I can feel your love like the warmth of the sun on my skin every day.

Tova, I admire your bravery, your adventurous spirit, and your creative soul. Growing up with you as my sister was the best part of my childhood.

Grandma, you are my role model. I hope to be as strong and resourceful and wise as you one day.

Sigge, you are a dog so you probably won't read this but you are serotonin in gift wrap.

Thank you John for holding my hand through the wonders and horrors of life, you feel like coming home. There's nobody else like you. I love you endlessly.

Thank you to my friends for all the fun we have! There's no others I'd rather stumble through my twenties alongside. Especially Nora and Linnea, because we've really gone through it together and cried a lot in front of each other.

My mentors Nadia, Suzanne and Kurt, who believed in me when I didn't. Teachers like you are like buoys to students who struggled to stay afloat.

This wouldn't have been possible without the wonderful team at Ebury and everyone who helped make this book materialize, huge thank you to lovely Leah, Faith, Sophie, Anya. My dream team!

And finally, to the people who built an online community with me, where we can be vulnerable, which is my favourite thing to be.

BIOGRAPHY

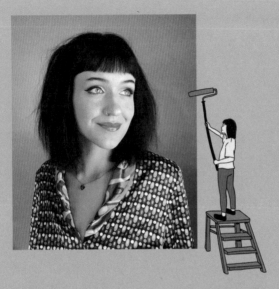

Matilda Heindow is an artist and mental health advocate based in Stockholm.

She founded the much-loved Instagram page @crazyheadcomics, using it as a creative outlet for her colourful cartoons that cleverly skewer our collective experiences of mental health. She has shared over 700 unique pieces of art to her global following and her work is often used by mental health professionals and schools.

In 2021, Matilda delivered a TEDx talk on 'The Art of Mental Health Advocacy'.